THE
ENERGY
EQUATION

FROM THE NAKED APE TO THE KNACKERED* APE

*Throughout this book, we are using the word 'knackered' in the British English slang meaning of the word, namely exhausted, worn out, or broken. No offence is intended to any person by such usage.

'There are one hundred and ninety three living
species of monkeys and apes. One hundred
and ninety-two of them are covered with hair.
The exception is the naked ape self-named Homo sapiens'

Desmond Morris,
Introduction to *The Naked Ape*,*1967

---

* For those of our lovely readers who are not old enough to have seen the book, *The Naked Ape : A Zoologist's Study of the Human Animal*, on every coffee table in every lounge, then here is a little background. Desmond Morris (1928 –) published this book in 1967. It was serialised in the *Daily Mirror* (thereby helping Craig's father's fledging newspaper business at the time!) and has been translated into 23 languages. Morris shows how human behaviour can be seen as evolved to meet the challenges of prehistoric life as a hunter. This idea fits well with the premise of this book – that we, Naked Apes, have become Knackered Apes because we are throwing away all the advantages that becoming the Naked Ape gave us, and that in the process, we have forgotten how to live and what to eat. In essence, our modern way of living is damaging to us, physically, cognitively and emotionally.

THE
ENERGY
EQUATION

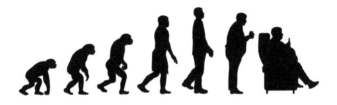

FROM THE NAKED APE TO
THE KNACKERED APE

DR SARAH MYHILL
AND CRAIG ROBINSON

BOOKS

Hammersmith Health Books
London, UK

First published in 2021 by Hammersmith Health Books
– an imprint of Hammersmith Books Limited
4/4A Bloomsbury Square, London WC1A 2RP, UK
www.hammersmithbooks.co.uk

British Library Cataloguing in Publication Data: A CIP record of this book is
available from the British Library.

Print ISBN 978-1-78161-185-2
Ebook ISBN 978-1-78161-186-9

Commissioning editor: Georgina Bentliff
Designed and typeset by: Sylvia Kwan
Cover design and chapter openers by: Madeline Meckiffe
Index: Dr Laurence Errington
Production: Helen Whitehorn, Pathmedia
Printed and bound by: TJ Books Ltd, Cornwall, UK

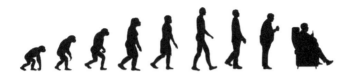

CONTENTS

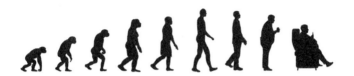

ABOUT THE AUTHORS

Dr Sarah Myhill MB BS qualified in medicine (with Honours) from Middlesex Hospital Medical School in 1981 and has since focused tirelessly on identifying and treating the underlying causes of health problems, especially the 'diseases of civilisation' with which we are beset in the West. She has worked in the NHS and private practice and for 17 years was the Honorary Secretary of the British Society for Ecological Medicine, which focuses on the causes of disease and treating through diet, supplements and avoiding toxic stress. She helps to run and lectures at the Society's training courses and also lectures regularly on organophosphate poisoning, the problems of silicone, and chronic fatigue syndrome. Visit her website at www.drmyhill.co.uk

Craig Robinson MA took a first in Mathematics at Oxford University in 1985. He then joined Price Waterhouse and qualified as a Chartered Accountant in 1988, after which he worked as a lecturer in the private sector, and also in the City of London, primarily in Financial Sector Regulation roles. Craig first met Sarah in 2001, as a patient for the treatment of his CFS/ME, and since then they have developed a professional working relationship, where he helps with the maintenance of www.drmyhill.co.uk, the moderating of Dr Myhill's Facebook groups and other ad hoc projects, as well as with the editing and writing of her books.

Stylistic note: Use of the first person singular in this book refers to me, Dr Sarah Myhill. One can assume that the medicine and biochemistry are mine, as edited by Craig Robinson and that the classical and mathematical references are Craig's.

'*You never change things by fighting the existing reality.*
To change something, build a new model that makes the
existing model obsolete'

Buckminster Fuller

Dedication

SM: To my lovely patients, who have been willing guinea pigs, faithful to the cause and most forgiving when my suggestions have not worked. However, in doing so, they have pushed forward the frontiers of ecological medicine.

CR: To all those men who have ever been saved and made into a better man by the presence in their lives of an extraordinary woman. And yes, I have just dedicated this book to myself. And yes, the extraordinary woman in question is you, Penny, the love of my life.

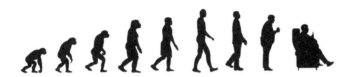

PREFACE

What determines the survival of the fittest is energy. Those animals with the most energy will be better feeders, movers and procreators. They will pass their energetic genes and survival strategies down to the next generation.

From hairy great apes, evolution has produced the super-successful, super-fit, clever calculating machines of us – the naked little apes. Modern homo sapiens should be fitter, stronger and cleverer than all previous versions. But we naked apes have become knackered apes. Physical, mental and emotional fatigues abound and these are the forerunners of obesity, diabetes, dementia, cancer and coronaries. Why?

The Energy Equation explains. It describes how to maximise energy delivery mechanisms in the body and then how to spend this energy efficiently by reducing immunological and emotional holes in your personal energy bucket and minimise energy-draining biochemical and mechanical frictions. Reducing and minimising these holes and frictions not only improves your own energy equation now, but also addresses the downstream effects of these holes and frictions – namely, the serious pathologies of the Western World.

This leaves us with an abundance of energy to spend on life, creating a safe ecological niche for our families, having fun, being creative and avoiding the dread diseases of our age.

Thus we can live to our full potential. Energy gives us quality and quantity of Life. Just do it.

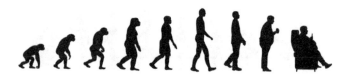

INTRODUCTION

I have spent most of my medical life looking to identify and treat the root causes of chronic fatigue syndrome. For these unfortunate patients, fatigue is pathological, severe, unrelenting and life changing. What has become clear through my personal medical evolution is that we can all benefit from those very same interventions that allow these patients to recover. This book is about how to recognise that we are not functioning to our full potential, why that is happening and so drive the intellectual imperative to change. These changes are within the grasp of us all. Once tackled and achieved you will not look back.

If you do not change direction, you may
end up where you are heading

Lao Tzu

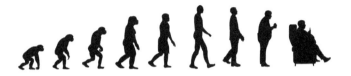

PART
1

THE KNACKERED APE

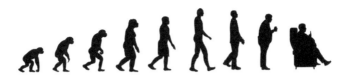

CHAPTER
1

THE NAÏVE DOCTOR STUMBLES
INTO THE REAL WORLD

I imagined becoming a doctor would be like being a mathematician – there would be interesting enigmas with a right answer and patients who'd live happily ever after in their solved state. Scientifically speaking, this should be possible.* If we could master all the schools of science and apply these specifically to each individual, we should see a satisfying result in all cases.

I left medical school on an intellectual high having qualified with honours. I felt I could face any patient with any problem and point them to a cure. This high was short lived. I quickly found out that medical education did little to prepare me for General Practice. Patients did not turn up with classic presentations of disease – indeed,

*Mathematical note by Craig: Mathematicians once made the assertion that everything that was true would have a mathematical proof. Gödel (logician and mathematician, 1906 – 1978) proved his so-called 'Incompleteness theorems' and in so doing threw that assertion out of the window. Sometimes true things cannot be proved. (This is a much-simplified version – interested Naked Apes can do their own research!)

such an occurrence was a rarity. They arrived with rheumatics, elusive headaches, malaises, and one, with his delightful Nottinghamshire accent 'am going down t' bank'. My fall-back position was to say that a blood test was needed and whilst awaiting the test results, I would anxiously leaf through my lecture notes or ask colleagues. Yes, this Naked Ape did not have the option of the Internet in those days. Only rarely did a clear answer present itself. Sometimes I would see the patient again and 'impress' them with the scholarly opine, 'It's a virus, variety: snuffly cold'. I might add in some complicated name for 'snuffly cold', such as 'rhinovirus' just for good measure. But by this time, they'd probably shaken off the 'snuffly cold'. Anyway, I soon found out that medics had a mediocre reputation, best iterated by Tolstoy (Russian author of *War and Peace*, 1828-1910): '*Though the doctors treated him, let his blood, and gave him medications to drink, he nevertheless recovered.*'

It wasn't an auspicious beginning, but it was to become much worse when I couldn't find any answers whatsoever for the 'tired all the time' patient. There were no obvious armpit boils, no yellow faces, no peculiar spine curvatures or other such helpful pointers. Indeed, these patients looked distressingly normal. They were direct, intelligent and sincere. They looked at me straight in the eye expecting a rational explanation. Many held down-high powered, responsible jobs, some had been high-achieving athletes. When tests returned with normal results, it was very tempting to give an airy wave of the hand and blame the problem on age, the menopause, idleness or hypochondria. But I lacked the gravitas necessary for such a conjuring act. I was forced onto the defensive. I had to admit that I did not know what on earth was going wrong. Even worse than that, I had to admit that I myself experienced some of the symptoms my patients were describing, and I too had no idea of the cause. This was in spite of six years of expensive, intensive and supposedly scientific medical education.

'Could it be something I am eating doc?' My immediate reaction was 'No'. I come from a long line of doctors, with my grandmother being one of the first women doctors in the UK, qualifying in 1922. Grandfather was senior registrar at Great Ormond Street under Sir George Frederic Stills, who described juvenile rheumatoid arthritis in children. My father and uncle were GPs. The dinner table conversation through childhood often dwelt on medical subjects and even before medical school I had a pretty good grasp of the major pathologies. Yes, I'd heard the very rare stories of peanuts causing acute collapse, but nowhere had the subject of food as a cause of chronic symptoms been aired. I even recall my father rubbishing a conversation with a family friend who maintained that a change of diet had allowed him to feel better. Father's diagnosis was 'deluded'. He had a reputation for being a good diagnostician so if he, all my other medical relatives and education determined that diet was irrelevant to pathology, then so it was.

Some Naked Apes, however, had made the connection that diet was important. In the 1920s, the nutritionist Victor Lindlahr was a strong believer in the idea that food directly affected health. That view gained some adherents and the earliest known printed example of his followers expressing this can be seen from an advert for beef in a 1923 edition of the *Bridgeport Telegraph*, for 'United Meet [sic] Markets': '*Ninety per cent of the diseases known to man are caused by cheap foodstuffs. You are what you eat.*'

There is something about medical training which starts with intelligent, enthusiastic and caring young students and turns them into narrow minded, arrogant and emotionless physicians.

They have the intelligence educated out of them.

Anon

This is further encouraged by the development of a language to prevent the patient from understanding and answering back. A wag of a registrar at the Middlesex Hospital London, where I trained, explained to us that dermatology is the art of choosing an unpronounceable name and then slapping on a steroid antimicrobial cream. Fungal infection of the penis is called *balanitis xerotica obliterans* or *lichen sclerosus et atrophicus*; smelly infected armpits are called *hidradenitis suppurativa*; heat rash is *milaria rubra*. But this is not diagnosis – this is a clinical picture. In looking at the stars, our distant Naked-Ape ancestors linked them together into familiar shapes and gave them Latin names like Aquarius, Capricornus and Ursa Major. But this is not science either – we call this astrology. I soon discovered that my patients were more incisive than I was. They were looking for the root cause of their symptoms. They were not content with an astrological clinical picture – they expected real science and the application of such. They did not want to consult an astrologist; they wanted a logical explanation for their constellation of symptoms from an astronomer. And I was found wanting at the first hurdle.

One of the early lessons I learned was that I was practising medicine in a lovely and forgiving community. They did not mind that I did not know the answer; they were very happy with me not knowing and saying so. They were happy that I could rule out serious illness, accept their suggestions for progress (because I did not have any of my own) and also, they were prepared to be willing guinea-pigs. And then, in the midst of these agonies and ignorance, occurred a life-changing experience.

Ruth was born. She, of course, was going to be the perfect baby, breast-fed and expertly managed by this highly qualified doctor recently furnished with the best of medical educations from one of the top London teaching hospitals. Within a few days of birth Ruth started howling and crying. Inconsolably. Nothing I could do made one jot of difference. Nothing anyone else could do made one jot of difference either. Various nostrums were recommended, including gripe water (alcohol), Calpol (paracetamol and sugar) and mebeverine (atropine like), but even at that stage of my education I knew this was symptom suppression. 'Oh Ducky, it's only three-month colic – it will pass.' I was suddenly aware that I was on the receiving end as a patient being fed astrology when I needed astronomy. I recall my then-husband Nick, overwhelmed by the screams, saying 'You're the effing doctor – you sort it out'. These days and nights were turning into the most miserable, confidence-sapping weeks of my life. I was exhausted, embarrassed by my inadequacy and had no idea what was going on.

At that point in time I would have been the ideal subject for any old Quack wielding snake oil – happy to try dancing naked at midnight with vestal virgins if there was a promise of a cure. Perhaps it was that memory of my father's 'deluded' diagnosis of the 'change-of-diet friend' that prompted me to think of food? Instinctively I cut out all dairy products. This was not easy because I loved them. I adored my milky drinks, my butter with my bread, my hunks of cheese and lashings of cream over puddings. But the results were miraculous. Within 36 hours Ruth slept longer than two hours. Then six hours. On one occasion when I was too shy to refuse a cup of tea to which milk had already been added she was up again screaming all night.

There were unforeseen benefits for me too. I had wheezed and sneezed my way through childhood. A considerable diagnostic breakthrough occurred when Father realised that his horse-allergic daughter was sleeping on a horsehair mattress! But cutting out dairy was a further transformation – for the first time I could leave the house without checking I had my snot rag to hand. Food had flavours previously unrecognised. These observations amounted to a miracle – but where was this information in those medical textbooks? Why was this not standard teaching? I realised a whole new area of medicine was opening up to me.

On the back of this crumb of knowledge I opened the Sherwood Allergy Clinic. I still wake in the night cringing at the childlike naivety with which I confidently faced patients. I only had one tool to play with – a diet that eliminated dairy products and grains. There were a few success stories, but I vividly recall one patient with multiple symptoms. As I launched into details of the diet she sighed. Yes, she had done all that without result so what next? She had bottomed the pit of my knowledge. I needed more tools.

That was the start of my uncomfortable journey into Ecological Medicine – the business of asking the question why? Nowhere were there more questions than from those patients suffering from chronic fatigue syndrome and ME. That was to become my area of special interest. The answers I found not only cured some and greatly improved many but were applicable to us all. Those answers allowed top athletes to improve their performance and normal people to function to their full potential. They have been life-changing for me personally and professionally.

So, let's fast forward to 2021, look back with the eye of experience and read on….

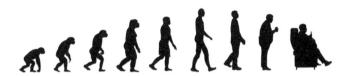

CHAPTER
2

FROM THE NAKED APE TO
THE KNACKERED APE

Energy is one of the most powerful survival forces. With energy one can run down any prey and harvest all day. With energy the brain thinks clearly, reacts quickly and makes good decisions to problem solve, foresee or escape trouble. Energy we perceive as a thing of beauty – we see it in our faces and movements. It attracts others to us. Energy allows us to procreate and survive tough times. Primitive man needed energy in abundance to survive an unforgiving environment.

So why is it that with our 'fabulous' system of food delivery and highly sophisticated infra-structures, fatigue is so common? We are better fed, watered, warmed, protected and entertained than ever before – we should be overflowing with energy! Hairy apes evolved into naked apes – active, intelligent and sociable. We now have knackered apes – fatigued, foggy and lonely. What happened?

'*George, where did it all go wrong?*' the caviar- and champagne-delivering waiter is reported to have said to the once brilliant footballer George Best, who was lying on his 5-star hotel room bed, strewn with fifty-pound notes, with the then current Miss World lying next to him.

The Energy Equation

The waiter was referring, of course, to George's 'early retirement'. Indeed, where did it go wrong for us all?

The Knackered Ape

I blame the doctors.

Fatigue may be the commonest medical symptom, but it is the worst treated by Western medicine. Doctors view fatigue as part of ageing and idleness when actually it is an early warning symptom of serious pathology. The root causes of fatigue are the same as those causes of serious illness. By misunderstanding and ignoring fatigue, doctors are failing to prevent cancer, coronaries, diabetes, dementia and degeneration.

The problem is that Western medicine no longer looks for disease causation. Arthritis, indigestion and depression are treated as deficiency disorders of prescription drugs, whose acronyms are NSAIDs, PPIs and SSRIs respectively. So, if a person suffers from depression then the Western doctor prescribes selective serotonin re-uptake inhibitors (SSRIs, such as Prozac) rather than look for the underlying causes of the depression. Finding those underlying causes will result in actual treatment and cure of the depression rather than merely suppressing the symptom. Such symptom suppression does not cure the pathology, but it is even worse than that – often these prescription drugs escalate disease processes. Actually, depression is effectively treated by tipping the energy equation in our favour.

So, these essential symptoms are red flags that warn us of impending pathology. Unpleasant symptoms should drive us on to make the necessary changes to relieve those symptoms and also to correct the underlying causes. If we suppress symptoms instead, then the disease process is accelerated. If 'treated' by modern Western symptom-suppressing medications, then arthritis leads to wheelchairs, indigestion to cancer and depression to suicide, which is now the commonest cause of death in young men.

Let's look at a clinical example – if a patient presented to a conventional doctor with an injury to his foot, first he would be prescribed painkillers. As the lesion failed to heal then antibiotics would be dished out and the patient would be given a stick to help him walk. However, gangrene might well set in and an amputation would result. By contrast, the ecological doctor, interested in root causes, would enquire about walking and foot wear. The nail in the shoe would be diagnosed and the patient cured.

I arrived at these views through my work with patients suffering from chronic fatigue syndrome (CFS) (pure pathological fatigue) and myalgic encephalitis (ME). (ME is CFS plus inflammation.) Both my patients and I have been subject to modern persecution for holding the apparently heretical view that the symptom of fatigue has physical causes and that there are effective physical treatments for it. My patients have been systematically abused by psychiatrists who insist that they are idle and deluded and that their symptoms are either 'imagined', or that their illnesses are in some way 'their fault'; this results in treatment with exercise and cognitive behaviour therapy. The psychiatrists' mantra has been that these patients can 'exercise' their way back to health and that their symptoms result merely from deconditioning and a 'false illness belief'. There is a plethora of medical studies showing serious pathology in CFS and ME patients and it is intellectually idle and risible to suggest that exercise is a 'cure'. Indeed, far from being a cure, this kind of 'treatment' can render the patient even more ill than before. Craig, an ME sufferer, spent more than four years bedridden after a nine-month course of cognitive behaviour therapy.

For my part, I have been continuously investigated and prosecuted by the General Medical Council (GMC) since 2001. This has occurred despite no patient ever having complained, no patient ever having been harmed and no patient ever having been put at risk of harm. I am now the most investigated doctor in the history of the GMC. I have been investigated 38 times and each time the GMC has dropped its proceedings against me with no case to answer. The score is currently Me 38: GMC 0. Apparently, what I am damaging is the reputation of the medical profession because I challenge the perceived wisdom, diagnose rather than suppress symptoms, and refuse to follow 'Guidelines' that I know are not in the best interests of my patients.

As was noted by a GMC legal opinion in an internal GMC memo dated 10th February 2006, during a concerted GMC attempt to obtain patient testimony against me: 'My main concerns with all the Myhill files are that all of the patients appear to be improving and none of them are likely to give WS (witness statements) or have complained about their treatment.' So, it was a 'problem' for the GMC that my patients were all improving and not willing to complain about me.

Even so, when I argued my case 'too strongly' at my GMC Interim Orders Panel Hearing in October 2010 I was suspended from the Medical Register because I 'lacked respect for my regulatory body, the GMC'. I could only be grateful that I had not lived 500 years previously or I would surely have been burned at the stake as a heretic. At least the modern (GMC) decision to suspend me was reversible, and indeed it was so reversed eight weeks later.

As the 18th-century French author Voltaire mused in *The Age of Louis XIV* '*It is dangerous to be right in matters on which the established authorities are wrong*.' Voltaire was correct in his assertion, but this should not deter us from following what we know to be the right path, and this applies to health, today even more than ever.

So, you are about to hear the views of a modern, medical heretic. I do not pretend to know all the answers, but I am at least asking the right questions. I believe that I do have enough of the right answers both to keep the healthy fighting fit and to reverse disease progression in the unwell.

I certainly know enough to point my CFS and ME patients in the right direction and give them the 'rules of the game' and the 'tools of the trade' to heal themselves. However, what is so interesting is that these rules and tools apply to us all. So much of what we must do to stay well and prevent illness boils down to the Energy Equation and there is so much that can be done to tip this equation in our favour.

Do it now, do it well. You can then spend your energy on fun and look forward to a life of quality and quantity. Just do it.

Do it or don't do it, There is no try.

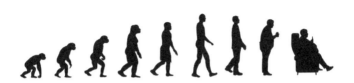

CHAPTER
3

THE KNACKEROMETER

What follows in this chapter is a way of measuring just how knackered ('exhausted' for my non-British readers) you are. You probably 'know' how bad (or perhaps even good!) things are already, but sometimes we Naked Apes need a little encouragement to convert from a state of knowing to a state of 'really knowing' and then to a state of doing.

Measuring can be a very useful tool, as long as it is done honestly, so, please approach this chapter with complete candour and do not try to hide the truth – you will only be hiding it from yourself.

Measurement is the first step that leads to control and eventually to improvement. If you can't measure something, you can't understand it. If you can't understand it, you can't control it. If you can't control it, you can't improve it.

H James Harrington, IBM quality expert, 1929 –

Our knackerometer measuring scale is subjective and relies on 'symptoms'.

Symptoms of low energy

We need to look at the symptoms that warn us that we are not generating enough energy and/or are spending too much.

My most precious possession is energy. I love spending it. I spend it physically trotting off with my terrier Nancy and grubbing in my garden; emotionally with my darling daughters; and mentally in problem solving with patients. To spend energy so joyfully I need a large and full bucket of the stuff. That means I must maintain a generous gap between energy delivery mechanisms and energy spending. I must stay in positive equity. Mr Micawber's famous, and oft-quoted, recipe for happiness is:

> *Annual income twenty pounds, annual expenditure nineteen*
> *[pounds] nineteen [shillings] and six [pence], result happiness.*
> *Annual income twenty pounds, annual expenditure twenty*
> *pounds ought and six, result misery.*

From *David Copperfield* by Charles Dickens (1812 – 1870)

In Life there is no such thing as negative equity. If energy spending exceeds delivery, cell function slows, organs fail and we die. We are protected from death by symptoms. A narrowing energy gap is a very risky business and so the brain generates deeply unpleasant symptoms to alert us, to stop us spending energy and so to prevent 'negative equity' (death). These nasty symptoms slow energy expenditure by the body, and by the brain and the immune system. Ask yourself if you experience, or suffer from, any of the issues listed in Table 3.1; these are the body's warning signs that your personal Energy Equation is edging towards negative equity. Ignore them at your peril!

Table 3.1: Symptoms of failing energy

Symptom	How this symptom prevents us spending energy (much more about mechanisms later)	Tick this box if you experience this
Physical fatigue	Stops us spending the energy we have not got; we slow down and rest up	
Mental fatigue	The brain weighs 2% of body weight but consumes 20% of total body energy production. If energy delivery is impaired, nerve conduction is slowed. Mental processing slows and so multi-tasking, problem-solving and much else decline. This is the starting point of brain failure or dementia, now the commonest cause of death in Westerners	
Pain	When energy delivery mechanisms are impaired the body switches into anaerobic metabolism. In the very short term this generates a little extra energy but at the price of lactic acid production. Lactic acid burn in muscles is very painful; it prevents gold medals being won	
Chest pain	Lactic acid burn in the heart results in the symptom of angina	
Deeply unpleasant mental symptoms such as:	The brain cannot and does not perceive pain, so it has to manifest with other symptoms to slow us down. It is biologically plausible that lactic acid burn and/or lack of the energy molecule ATP, in the brain, drive other nasty symptoms such as:	
– feeling stressed	This deeply unpleasant symptom arises when the brain knows it does not have the reserves to deal with demands. It drives us to major strategic lifestyle, energy-conserving changes, such as selling houses and ditching spouses	
– feeling depressed	This makes us antisocial (social interactions are demanding of energy). The depressed patient wants to be left alone, curl up in a corner and be miserable. We all feel a bit like this in the winter and this represents a primitive drive to conserve energy and so survive the winter. Being happy is great fun but costs energy	

Table 3.1: Symptoms of failing energy (cont.)

Symptom	How this symptom prevents us spending energy (much more about mechanisms later)	Tick this box if you experience this
– feeling anxious	This is the symptom the brain generates when it believes it will not have the energy to deal with demands	
– being angry and irritable	This inhibits others from making demands of us	
– looking tired and stressed, appearing angry and anxious	The face is the mirror of the mind, reflecting precisely our precious energy stores. Facial expression allows others to see our energy reserves – another essential survival technique	
Using social addictions to cope	Addictions mask symptoms. This is dangerous practice. Symptoms protect us from ourselves. Addictions give us the temporary and false impression that all is well. But as the dose diminishes, the devil returns, until of course we take another dose of our addiction. The obvious addictions are to 'illegal' and 'legal highs', such as cocaine, speed, nicotine, caffeine and alcohol, but the worst addiction in terms of morbidity and mortality is to sugars and starches. Once recognised as such, much pathology of Westerners is explained, and this starts with fatigue	
Using prescription drug addictions to cope	Psychiatrists have yet to wake up to the fact that most mental disorders start with poor energy equity which is followed by masking with addiction. Most drugs for psychological conditions add to this addictive load with the usual short-term gain, long-term pain outcome	
Energy-saving behavioural changes	Procrastination, going slow, choosing energy-saving tools – such as riding rather than walking. I was upset recently by the sight of a spherical child on an electric scooter	

Pick up every cough, cold and tummy bug	The immune system, when activated to fight, consumes much energy	
Poor libido	The business of procreation, in all its phases, is hugely demanding of energy. If this is lacking, babies will not survive	
Poor posture	Standing correctly requires muscle power to keep us straight – which needs energy. As we run out of energy, we curl up and this starts with stooping.	

So, how do you know if you have good energy delivery mechanisms? Remember we have no objective measures of the state of the energy bucket – it is all about symptoms. Table 3.2 lists the indicators of a healthily full energy bucket.

If there are no ticks in Table 3.1 and no crosses in Table 3.2, shut this book, slap it on the table and shoot off for some fun. After that, maybe drop this manual for good health into your local library in the hope that a Knackered Ape may spot it, even perhaps the librarian. However, if ticks and crosses there be or, worse still, if the ticks and crosses abound, then your knackerometer reading is too high and, Dear Reader, you must read on.

Table 3.2: Indications that your energy balance is tipped in your favour

Mechanism	Symptom	Put a cross in this box if this is NOT true for you
Good energy delivery to the body	Wake naturally, feeling on top of the world Have lots of energy to spend on doing things Feel well even at the end of a busy day	
Good energy delivery to the brain...	Feel confident, optimistic, easy-going, relaxed, patient, generous, sociable	
	Accept criticism	
	Feel nothing is too much trouble	
	Have a good sense of humour	
	Are quick witted	
	Make good decisions	
	Give love freely and without conditions attached	
	Are altruistic	
	Always have a new horizon, new interest or hobby	
...which is reflected in the face	Smile and laugh	
	Look 'attractive', possibly even 'beautiful'	
...and actions	Sing, whistle or hum	
	Walk with a spring in the step	
	Have expansive body language	
Good energy delivery to the immune system	Resist all infection! When all around are going down with some ghastly bug you are left standing.	

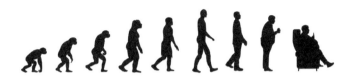

CHAPTER
4

THE ENERGY EQUATION

First and most important is to understand the road map. *Again* I quote Mr Micawber's recipe for happiness from *David Copperfield* by Charles Dickens: '*Annual income twenty pounds, annual expenditure nineteen [pounds] nineteen [shillings] and six [pence], result happiness. Annual income twenty pounds, annual expenditure twenty pounds ought and six, result misery.*'*

And so it is with energy. We have to look at both sides of the equation – how the body generates energy and how it is spent. As Mr Micawber so brilliantly points out, if we get it right, then the result is happiness. In this sense, energy is like money – it is great fun spending it and jolly hard work earning it. And what is more important than happiness? Audrey Hepburn (1929-1993) knew this: '*The most important thing is to enjoy your life – to be happy – it's all that matters.*'

***Footnote:** Charles Dickens (1812 – 1870) wrote *The Personal History, Adventures, Experience and Observation of David Copperfield the Younger of Blunderstone Rookery* in 1849. For those with no knowledge of pre-decimal British currency, there were 12 pennies in a shilling (5 p at the time of decimalisation in 1971) and 20 shillings to the pound. Hence the difference between happiness and misery is very small but highly significant.

The Energy Equation

How the body generates energy for life

The word 'doctor' comes from the Latin *docere*, 'to teach'. My job is to teach my patients how to cure themselves. I have to distil 60 years of learning into a 60-minute consultation to be effective. To achieve a clinical result, the messages I carry must be comprehensible, logical, persuasive and memorable. To this end, analogies are very useful and one that has stood the test of time to explain energy generation is the comparison with a car.

Figure 4.1 – Car-energy analogy
Energy delivery in the body – think of the body as a car

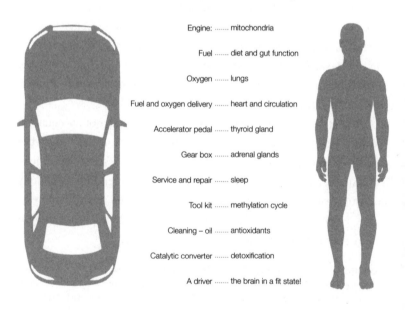

Engine: .... mitochondria

Fuel .... diet and gut function

Oxygen .... lungs

Fuel and oxygen delivery .... heart and circulation

Accelerator pedal .... thyroid gland

Gear box .... adrenal glands

Service and repair .... sleep

Tool kit .... methylation cycle

Cleaning – oil .... antioxidants

Catalytic converter .... detoxification

A driver .... the brain in a fit state!

For our car to run there are four important players: the correct fuel in the tank, an engine to burn that fuel, then an accelerator pedal and gear box to match energy demand to energy delivery. The body is the same but the names different. For fuel read food, for engine read mitochondria, leaving us with the thyroid accelerator pedal and the adrenal gear box. Finally, we need to service and repair our engines during sleep. If we concentrate our attention on these fundamentals, not only do we energise ourselves, but we extend lifespans and prevent all of the diseases associated with Western lifestyles.[†]

The above functional unit is common to all animals from slugs and snails to puppy dogs and quails. For many primitive animals the heart, lungs, circulation, kidneys and liver are absent, not being central to energy delivery mechanisms but they all need to make energy to spend it.

How the body spends energy

1. Basal metabolism

Your basal metabolism is the first priority; then you can have a life.

The business of simply staying alive, which is what we call 'basal metabolism', consumes two-thirds of all the energy generated by the body. After that, energy must be prioritised for activities that keep us and our genes alive: survival: food, shelter, security and lastly procreation. Any left over after that can then be spent having a life. Thank goodness I live in modern times where not all my energy is consumed by harvesting, building, fighting wars and keeping warm. Thank goodness too I have the spare energy to have some fun.

[†]**Note from Craig:** In a single paragraph Sarah has summed up the essence of both how to be healthy and how to stay healthy. Read on for the detail. Diet (page 147); Mitochondria (page 49); Thyroid (page 57); Adrenals (page 57) Sleep (page 67).

2. The immunological hole in the energy bucket

There are occasions when we must spend energy to deal with the unexpected. Acute infection – and this would have been a big killer for our Fred and Wilma Flintstones – demands an effective armed response from our standing army, the immune system. Armies need energy in abundance to run a fever because heat kills all microbes. Our white cell soldiers need ammunition and the power to fire cytokine bullets and lob interleukin grenades at our infectious invaders. During such an onslaught, Fred would curl up in the back of his cave away from predators, wrap up in a warm nest and lie still until his immunological army had won the battle. His brain would have given him symptoms of acute fatigue, causing illness behaviour, so that energy could be diverted to fight the good fight. Meanwhile, Wilma would have gone off hunting, picked berries, looked after the children and consoled Fred in his misery.

The problem with our modern world is that the immune system gets switched on inappropriately, resulting in allergy and autoimmunity.

- Allergy is the inflammation which results from responses to substances (called 'antigens') from outside the body.

- Autoimmunity is the inflammation that results from responses to tissues within the body.

We are seeing epidemics of both. We are fighting the bad fight, and this is kicking a hole in our energy bucket. In Chapter 12 we look at how to deal with the immunological hole in the energy bucket.

3. The emotional hole in the energy bucket – the brain

Although the brain accounts for just 2% of total body weight, it consumes 20% of all energy generated. This fact alone illustrates the survival value to a species conferred by a brain – we value it so highly that we pour energy into it. Brains define cultivation and culture, society and socialisation. They are what it is to be human and humane – the most complex, fascinating, divine creation of our known universe. But energy can be wasted by the brain. Being stressed or anxious in the short term may confer survival value but long-term, unremitting stress and anxiety waste energy and shorten life.

The key to a fun and productive life

The key to a fun and productive life is therefore to get the Energy Equation right by maximising energy delivery and making energy expenditure as efficient as possible by doing the following:

Improving energy delivery mechanisms: Energy *in*

- Sort out the engine and control mechanisms (see Chapters 5 to 9)
- Optimise energy delivery through exercise (see Chapter 10)
- Make the most of free energy – something for nothing (see Chapter 11)

Managing energy expenditure: Energy *out*

- Minimise expenditure on your basal metabolism (see Chapter 12)
- Attend to the immunological hole in your store of energy – what I call the 'energy bucket' (see Chapter 13)
- Attend to the emotional hole in the energy bucket (see Chapter 14).

Thus, we have it, an equation for happiness!

For happiness we need our energy equation to be in surplus and the energy left over for happiness is exactly that surplus of the energy delivery over the energy expenditure, as described above:

Happiness = Energy Delivery MINUS Energy Expenditure

Personally, I prefer my equation for happiness to that developed by researchers at University College London, funded by the Wellcome Trust:

$$\textbf{Happiness}(t) = w_0 + w_1 \sum_{j=1}^{t} \gamma^{t-j}\, \textbf{CR}_j + w_2 \sum_{j=1}^{t} \gamma^{t-j}\, \textbf{EV}_j + w_3 \sum_{j=1}^{t} \gamma^{t-j}\, \textbf{RPE}_j$$

$$+ w_4 \sum_{j=1}^{t} \gamma^{t-j} \max\left(\textbf{R}_j - \textbf{O}_j, 0\right) + w_5 \sum_{j=1}^{t} \gamma^{t-j} \max\left(\textbf{O}_j - \textbf{R}_j, 0\right)$$

So, let's look at my equation for happiness in the rest of the book!

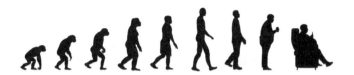

CHAPTER
5

THE KNACKERED APE
IS AN ADDICT

Remember the energy equation must be kept in positive equity. If energy demands exceed delivery, we die. To prevent this, the brain and body give us deeply unpleasant symptoms to stop us spending energy.

However, spending energy is fun! *Homo exhaustus* has discovered that he can mask those nasty symptoms with social, illegal and prescription drugs. Physical and mental fatigue can be masked by caffeine, speed (amphetamine), cocaine and ecstasy. Stress can be eliminated by opiates, cannabis, alcohol and nicotine. Anxiety can be masked by alcohol and carbohydrates. We call the latter 'comfort eating'. In Nottinghamshire when I was a GP there, the favourite comfort food was a chip butty. In Scotland it was a sugar sandwich, to be replaced more recently by a deep-fried Mars Bar. In the very short-term, eating such foods brings blood sugar up and there is a window of optimum levels for energy delivery mechanisms, but blood sugar levels that are too high or too low both result in fatigue. Many people with diabetes first go to their doctor with fatigue and a foggy brain. Indeed, dementia is now being called 'type III diabetes'.

A patient in denial

A memorable consultation was with Jim. It was immediately apparent that he was a successful and intelligent businessman and that I needed to match such to communicate effectively with him. My opening question therefore was 'What are your addictions?'. He was much taken aback and, without much thought, replied 'None'. Now, the most important part of any medical examination is the patient's 'history' and central to my history taking is finding out about diet and addiction. It became quickly apparent that there was little in Jim's daily life that was not addictive. The day started with coffee, orange juice and muesli with milk. Through the day the coffee continued but he also vaped (better than smoking but still an addiction). Lunch was often a business lunch with sandwiches and sometimes a beer. Tea and biscuits followed. In the evening he would have two glasses of wine with his supper of meat, potatoes rice or pasta followed by ice cream. Some evenings he smoked a joint. Occasionally for a business meeting, so as to appear energised and sharp, he used cocaine.

Jim truly believed he was not an addict because all those things he perceived as potentially being addictive he was using in moderation. Furthermore, he was complying with the, as you will discover risible, recommended five portions a day of fruit and vegetable. So that was okay then.

The addiction ladder

I see Western Life as a progression through addiction. It starts with the baby fed milk. All formula milks are high in sugar and baby guzzles them down, is satisfied for a few hours, but then the blood sugar level falls and s/he wakes screaming for more. The poor little mite is constantly stressed by the adrenalin of falling blood sugar which

> *My name is Craig and I was a crisp addict. I ate at least eight 'normal–sized' packets of ready-salted crisps a day. Sometimes I preferred the 'salt'n'shake' variety. See how I say, 'normal sized', as if I am still trying to let myself off. There is a lot of denial in addiction. I had stashes of crisps in the kitchen, in a cupboard in the shower room and in my bedroom wardrobe. I would sometimes wake up in the middle of the night and eat two packets, quietly so as not to wake my wife. Even writing about crisps sets off the saliva response. I gave up crisps in one single day about 10 years ago and I have never eaten a packet since then and I never will again, although I will always want to. Addiction is a very strong impulse. Be honest and accept your own addictions, and then deal with them! (PS: For 'at least eight' read 'about 10' – that was the addict in me speaking... .)*

disturbs sleep. By contrast, my friend Michelle ate a ketogenic (low-carb) diet throughout pregnancy and breast-feeding and weaned Baby Robyn on the same. The result? From a few days, Robyn slept through the night. By two months she was regularly sleeping from 7:00 pm to 8:00 am. She is the most contented, bright, bonny and happy baby. I expect her to have a very healthy life.

The addictive ladder starts with milk and sugar but often moves on to fruit as babies are weaned on banana, stewed apple and juice. Actually, fruit sugar is more pernicious than the white stuff and upsets blood sugar levels even more. (For the biochemists, this is because it inhibits the enzyme glycogen phosphorylase so that the liver cannot easily release sugar from glycogen as blood sugar levels fall). Most mothers are addicted and love to feed their children the foods they love. Chocolate is addictive. Coca-cola is addictive. As the child grows up, parents inevitably lose control. I have a rule of thumb that between the ages of 14 and 24 parents are so 'out of control of their children' that all they can do is cross their fingers and hope for the best.

Our Western child grows into a stressed world, made more so now by social media. S/he can easily access different drugs to control his stressful symptoms and so moves up the addictive ladder with nicotine, alcohol and cannabis. Remember that, in masking symptoms we become more attractive to others – we have false energy to dance all night, be witty, funny and extrovert. The poor teenager then has the double whammy of increasing life stress and withdrawal symptoms as the drug effect wears off. This often manifests with depression. Some kids simply progress up the additive ladder, moving on to hard drugs such as opiates or cocaine, to control their distressing symptoms. Some go to doctors for help, but only too often they are prescribed a further addiction – possibly a minor tranquiliser like Valium (diazepam) but sometimes, if there is any hint of psychosis, a major tranquilliser or antidepressant. Despite drug company protestations, even antidepressant drugs are addictive. The SSRI class of antidepressant ('selective serotonin re-uptake inhibitors') have a further danger of causing acute suicidal thinking and, indeed, suicide is the commonest cause of death in young men in the UK and Ireland.

Thankfully, the natural progression for most is that they recognise their serious addictions and struggle their way back down the addictive ladder. I have huge admiration and respect for those young people who have achieved such.

Jim quickly recognised his progress through the muddy waters of addiction. He saw how one addiction switched on craving for another. A trip to the pub for a beer triggered craving for a cigarette and then a high-carb snack. What I now know is that sugar and carbohydrates are the most pernicious addiction because:

- the physical harm they cause has yet to be appreciated
- they are cheap, convenient, widely available and instantly effective
- associated with love.

Think of the advertising propaganda associated with carbs:

'a Mars a day helps you work rest and play'...

'all because the lady loves Milk Tray'...

'the best thing since sliced bread'...

There is another interesting aspect of addiction which has to do with the rate of dosing. The heroin addict has to inject directly into the bloodstream to get his hit. The nicotine addict must inhale – nicotine hits the brain within seconds of doing so. The alcohol addict drinks quickly on an empty stomach to achieve his hit. I have noticed that the serious alcohol addict will sup his gin and inhale through the alcohol in his mouth so that he inhales alcohol and, like the smoker, can achieve a hit in seconds.

The serious carb addict achieves his hit in three ways. First, he eats carbs that can be rapidly absorbed without digestion. That is *anything* that tastes sweet. Secondly, he takes his carbs in a liquid form, such as fruit juice, 'pop' and other such, since the sugar is already dissolved – indeed, it can even be absorbed in the mouth. Thirdly, he gobbles his food without waiting to savour the flavour. This latter is an important point. So many patients tell me that they eat carbs because they 'like them'. They fail to analyse the reason for liking. Actually, the liking is for the addictive hit which comes in association with flavour.*

Artificial sweeteners are no replacement for sugar. The body is intelligent and quickly learns that a sweet flavour in the mouth will be followed by a sugar spike and releases insulin in anticipation of this, thereby triggering the same pernicious effects on energy delivery mechanisms.

I could see Jim's eyes glazing over as I launched into my addiction diatribe. At that point, little did he know that I would be asking him to give up all his addictions. In order of seriousness I considered these to be cocaine, fruit, sugar and carbs, alcohol, cannabis, nicotine and caffeine. For him to be able to achieve this he had to have the intellectual imperative to do so. I can be strong willed if I put my mind to something, but I have to have a jolly good reason because I, like other sane citizens, love a comfortable life.

So, did he do it? Eventually! It is a rare patient who kicks all their addictions over-night. Most have to come slowly down the addiction ladder and I now see that what slows progress is the sensation of bereavement as they say good-bye to their favourites. I now see better results when I address this issue directly. We associate having fun with addiction. Watching England play Rugby at Twickenham or England beat the Aussies at Lords has to be accompanied by a couple of pints. I do deals with my patients which amount to: *first* you must do whatever

---

*Note from Craig: This was so true of my addiction to crisps. Towards the end of my addiction, I was buying the cheapest variety going – in large packs of 20 packets. I really didn't care what they actually tasted like. I even justified my addiction by thinking that eating crisps was cheaper than eating other food types and so that in fact I was doing a good thing by eating crisps… . The addict's mind is very contrived. Sometimes I couldn't wait even to pay for the crisps and would eat a couple of packets before I got to the checkout. As I said above, please do think very hard and do not let yourself off the hook. If you read this chapter and think you may have an addiction, accept that fact and deal with it.

is necessary to realise your full potential; *then*, and only then, can you use addiction on the occasional basis to enhance a social situation.

Alcohol is a good servant but a poor master

Next let us explore what it is about a low-carb ketogenic diet that is so good for energy.

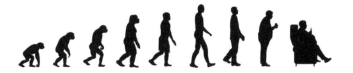

PART
2

ENERGY GENERATION

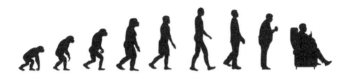

CHAPTER
6

HOW THE BODY GENERATES
ENERGY FOR LIFE

FIRST THE FUEL IN THE TANK

The Prussian ruler, Frederick the Great (1712 – 1786), is quoted as saying: 'T*he army marches on its stomach*'. He should have known; during his reign, expenditure on the army represented 86% of the total state budget and led to the saying: '*La Prusse n'est pas un pays qui a une armée, c'est une armée qui a un pays.*' – '*Prussia is not a country that has an army; it's an army that has a country*'.

Following the 1991 Gulf War, the USA army analysed the reasons for deaths by friendly fire. Front-line troops were told that during the initial advances they could not expect to be supported during the first five days – they had to carry all their supplies with them. Not surprisingly they loaded up with ammunition at the expense of food. But feeding the soldier is as vital as feeding the guns. Many of the deaths from friendly fire came from soldiers who were low on fuel (that is, food) and therefore energy. A poorly energised brain makes bad decisions and some of these troops made very bad decisions. Friendly fire deaths arose from these soldiers being half-starved.

In consequence, the US army asked Dr Keira Clarke of Oxford University to do some research to work out how soldiers could be most efficiently fuelled – to find something that they could carry and would supply the best weight to power ratio – that is, the lightest fuel for the greatest energy.

All food, from sugars and starches to protein and fat, has to be converted into ketone bodies before it can be used to fuel our mitochondrial engines. Perhaps feeding soldiers with ketones was a possibility? It so happened that the adjacent laboratory was researching ketones, and so she upgraded production to produce sufficient amounts to power a human for a day. She then tested her ketone drink on elite athletes – those runners and cyclists in full training at the peak of their careers. Could their performance be improved further by feeding them this ketone drink? As often occurs, scientists with a good idea hate to waste time on formal trials and ethical committee approval and simply test it, on the quiet, on themselves.

Scientists who experiment on themselves

Barry Marshall is the doctor who demonstrated that symptoms of indigestion and acidity might be due to an infection with the bacterium Helicobacter pylori. *He deliberately infected himself with such and suffered all the related symptoms. He then treated himself with antibiotics and was cured.*

Sometimes (applied) mathematicians do this too. Sir Isaac Newton, whilst studying optics, looked at the sun's reflection in a mirror for an extended period of time to see what would happen and was temporarily blinded in one eye. He suffered severe photophobia for a while and had to retreat to a darkened room for many days.

There are many more such examples.[1]

Dr Clarke was not an athlete, but her husband was a good middle-distance cyclist. Simply by drinking this ketone drink three times daily (and, yes, it tasted disgusting!) he was able to improve his performance, overnight, by 15%. Encouraged, she formally trialled the ketone drink and saw similar results in her elite Olympic athletes: they too improved performance by 7-15%. That makes the difference between a medal and an 'also ran'. I suspect, but do not know, that this helped Team GB to a record number of medals in the 2016 Olympics, knocking China into third place.

The ketone that Dr Clarke used was beta-Hydroxybutyric acid. This is the ketone that is normally produced in the body when the body is fuelled by fat and, indeed, we know that keto-adapted endurance athletes perform better than their carbohydrate-loaded peers. The world record for the furthest distance run in 24 hours is held by the keto-adapted Mick Morten, who covered 172 miles.

There is a further obvious reason why storing fuel as fat is helpful. Fat is a concentrated and dense fuel; by contrast, carbohydrates are stored as glycogen, which has an osmotic load and holds water. Consequently, the carb-loaded athlete will carry up to 2 kilograms of extra water and this immediately puts him at a power-weight disadvantage to his keto-adapted competitor. Finally, the keto-adapted athlete has a large pantry to draw upon – even the leanest male athlete is about 6-13% fat (women elite athletes, 14-20%) – but this supplies enough fuel to run 172 miles and much more. The carb-loaded athlete cannot go more than 17 miles without running out of fuel – the Americans call this 'bonking', the British 'hitting a wall'. It can be avoided by feeding the carb-loaded runner sweet drinks or gels – a ploy not available to front-line troops.

Ketones are as vital a fuel for the brain as for the body. Dementia is now the commonest cause of death in Westerners. Dr Dale Bredesen, a Californian neurologist, trialled a ketogenic diet in 10 patients with dementia and found an amazing change. The dementia was severe –

all had been forced to give up work; many needed care and would get lost in familiar surroundings; all had appalling short-term memory. To quote Dr Bredesen: 'The magnitude of improvement was unprecedented... In each of these cases, obvious subjective improvement, noted by the patient, his/her significant other and his/her co-workers, was accompanied by clear, quantitated, objective improvement. In the cases of patients 1 and 2, the improvement was of a magnitude not reported previously for patients with Alzheimer's disease. None of the 10 patients exhibited the cognitive decline that is characteristic of Alzheimer's disease, and the improvement experienced by all 10 has been sustained, with the longest time on the program being four years.'[2]

So, if ketones from eating fat and fibre are so obviously the preferred fuel for physical performance and mental sharpness, why do Westerners now eat more sugars and starches than ever before? Wherever any such debate exists I always go back to Nature and evolutionary principles for the answers.

The evolutionary principles

Humans are almost unique in their ability to run on two fuels. We can power our bodies with ketones (from fat and fibre) and with glucose (from sugar and starches). This affords huge evolutionary advantages since, if food availability changes with the seasons, climate or migration, humans can survive. Humans evolved as omnivorous hunter-gatherers. As we migrated away from the Equator we had to adjust to the seasons. This meant that during the winter, spring and much of the summer, we relied on hunting for meat, fish and shellfish as our staples. However, there would always be a natural autumn harvest of sugars and starches. Humans adapted to take advantage of this bonanza. Gorging on such foods made us fat and this conferred an essential survival advantage – fat for insulation and a pantry for the coming winter. There may have been an addiction gene that evolved in response to this natural harvest which drove us to eat those foods in an addictive way. Blood sugar spiked, insulin poured out to store that sugar as fat, blood sugar fell and made us hungry for more. We now call this biochemical state of affairs 'metabolic syndrome'. For short windows of time it conferred huge survival benefits. Now it is killing us because we are addicts who can access those addictive substances at all times (including during the night when we think of Craig's former crisp habit).

Metabolic syndrome

The modern western human (the Knackered Ape) is an addict and we pander to those addictions because we can. The primitive human simply ran out of addictive foods with the onset of winter; by contrast, the modern human has developed systems of agriculture, food storage and delivery which mean addictive foods and habits are not just a few pence but also a few minutes away. We recognise the delightful addictive potential of tobacco and alcohol, and governments tax them accordingly. We have yet to acknowledge that sugar and carbohydrates are equally addictive and equally pernicious, although the UK has introduced a 'sugar tax' of sorts – the Soft Drinks Industry Levy. Unfortunately this Levy is currently set at a level where it will raise tax income but not significantly change behaviour. Look at modern Western diets through the eyes of an addict and realise that, like any other addiction, we eat and snack to combat that nasty symptom we call stress. (Bear in mind, stress is a symptom the brain gives us to prevent us getting into negative energy equity – see page 57.) In the short term, eating addictive foods masks that symptom of stress and so gives us the false sensation of having energy. As the addictive hit wears off, we then experience withdrawal symptoms of stress with irritability and hunger and are driven to eat again. The addictive roller-coaster of a carbohydrate-based diet is the same as that of cocaine, morphine and cannabis: relief, withdrawal and craving.

Diagnosing metabolic syndrome: history, symptoms, signs, tests

Doctors' definition of metabolic syndrome is based on advanced symptoms, but diagnosis begins with looking at the contents of a person's supermarket trolley. Perhaps the most important aspect of any of my consultations relates to diet and identifying features of metabolic syndrome (and its inevitable results – namely diabetes, arterial disease, cancer and dementia) are as listed in Table 6.1.

Table 6.1: Do you have metabolic syndrome? Tick the box on the right if you have these symptoms and signs – the more ticks, the more trouble

	Question	Comments	Score: tick if yes to any of these
History	Which foods regularly appear in your shopping basket?	Staples: bread, potatoes, pulses, pasta, biscuits, pastry, fruit, cereals? Snacks: cereal bars, nut bars, sweets, crisps, chocolate, biscuits, cake, buns?	
	What do you eat for breakfast?	Cereal, porridge, toast, fruit juice, bagel, croissant?	
	Do you snack in the day...?	...on any of the above?	
	What do you drink in the day?	Anything other than water, black or green tea or coffee? Do you have pop, fruit juice, anything with artificial sweeteners?	

	Question	Comments	Score: tick if yes to any of these
	Would you suffer if you missed a snack or meal?		
	Do you need a sweet pudding to feel satisfied after your main meal?		
	Do you snack in the evening...	...on any of the above?	
Symptoms	Do you have any symptoms of fatigue...	...as detailed in Chapter 3 (page 16)?	
Signs	Are you overweight OR Do you struggle to lose weight?		
	Do you have dental disease?	Such as dental plaque, fillings, gum disease, tooth loss?	
	Is your jaw undershot?	You need to have or have had a dental brace, or been diagnosed with TMJ problems or poor bite (soft food means lack of chewing and so the jaw fails to develop)	
	Do you have 'man boobs'?		
Signs of fermenting gut	Do you suffer from indigestion, reflux or bloating?	See below	
	Are you apple shaped?	Beer bellies arise from the double whammy of high carbs and inoculation with yeast to ferment the carbs	

Table 6.1: Do you have metabolic syndrome? (cont.)

	Question	Comments	Score: tick if yes to any of these
	Do you suffer from joint or muscle pain? Do you take paracetamol or NSAIDs?	Arthritis is also part of metabolic syndrome – I suspect this is an inflammatory process driven by microbes from the carb-fermenting upper gut	
Tests	Blood pressure high: >140/90 mm Hg		
	Fasting triglycerides >1.5 mmol/l		
	Low proportion of HDL to total cholesterol	Easily calculated by dividing HDL by total cholesterol; the result should be >35%	
	Fasting blood sugar >6.0 mmol/l		
	Glycosylated haemoglobin >36 mmol/l		
	Ultrasound shows fatty liver		

How many ticks have you made? The more ticks, the more trouble as you will learn.

How to deny that you have metabolic syndrome

It is a feature of addiction that those most addicted develop the best rationalisations for such. If a patient starts to explain to me why they, in particular, cannot possibly be a carbohydrate addict, that increases the likelihood that I have made a correct diagnosis. (As I said, denial is a big part of addiction – Craig.) Table 6.2 lists the reasons I hear most often from patients to explain why they do not need to give up their high-carb diet and also my responses.

The evolutionarily correct diet is the Paleo-Ketogenic diet. Paleo means no dairy and no gluten grains; ketogenic means so that the body is powered by fat and fibre, not sugar and starch. All our energy delivery mechanisms evolved to run primarily on fat, and the human gut, brain, immune system, heart, muscles, liver further benefit.

Table 6.2: The commonest reasons my patients give not to change

The patient's reason	My response
I already eat a healthy balanced diet with my five-a-day fruit and vegetables	You have been well and truly brainwashed by industry propaganda. Your education starts here. Health is defined by outcomes – and you are on your way to disease and premature death. 'Balanced' is without definition and so meaningless Fruit is a 'bag of sugar'. Many vegetables are a 'bag of carbs'
But I have always eaten like this – why change now?	It takes decades of metabolic syndrome before pathology bites. Lao Tsu, author of *The Art of War,* wrote '*If you do not change direction you may end up where you are heading.*'
	Evolution is only interested in procreation – metabolic syndrome gets us that far then dumps us early on the evolutionary scrap heap, with cancer, heart disease and dementia. Nature does not care two hoots so long as the genetic Olympic flame has been passed on to the next generation
I wake late and have to leave for work so there is no time for anything other than a grabbed snack	Setting the alarm clock 30 minutes earlier is of proven benefit in improving sleep quality. Once established on the PK diet (see page 147), sleep improves further
I have no time to change my diet	Once established on the PK diet, you will only need two meals a day. You will not need to waste time on lunch and snacking
I have done the Atkins diet in the past and it did not work	The Atkins diet allows artificial sweeteners which maintain the sugar craving. It also allows dairy which is a common allergen

Table 6.2: The commonest reasons my patients give not to change (cont.)

The patient's reason	My response
I cannot prepare food for two different diets	If you really love your family, then they should all be eating PK! So should your dog and cat – meat, fish and eggs only please
I have tried this diet before and felt so ill that I could not carry on	That is a good sign – no addict can recover without going through withdrawal symptoms. Think of this as a healing crisis. If you really struggle to keto-adapt (see page 147), then you need our book *Ecological Medicine* as you may have a thyroid problem
I don't know what to eat	Read *The PK Cookbook* written by Yours Truly and Craig for precisely this reason
I just can't do it	If you do not do the PK diet, then really all other interventions are to no avail. The PK diet is non-negotiable. Do not waste my time (yes, I know that I am an angry, irritable old woman).

The upper fermenting gut

A further major problem for those running on carbs is the upper fermenting gut. The normal (I mean 'healthy', not 'usual') state of affairs in the gut is that the upper gut is near sterile for the business of digesting fat and protein whilst the lower gut is full of friendly bacteria to ferment fibre to short chain fats. However, if we eat so many carbs that we overwhelm the body's ability to digest and absorb them, microbes will move in to ferment them. The gastroenterologists call this 'small bowel bacterial overgrowth'. I call it' upper fermenting gut' because yeasts, as well as bacteria, are fermenters. Fermentation is just the chemical breakdown of a substance by bacteria, yeasts, or sometimes other microorganisms.*

The upper fermenting gut overloads the liver and poisons us in at least three ways:

1. Sugars are fermented into alcohols, noxious gases (ammonia and hydrogen sulphide) and peculiar sugars, such as D lactate.

2. Bacteria and fungi produce their own nasties in order to defend their microbial mini environment. We call these bacterial endotoxins and fungal mycotoxins.

3. The hydrogen sulphide of the fermenting gut combines with inorganic metals in food to convert them into easily absorbed organic metals. These 'bio-accumulate' in the heart, brain, kidneys and bone.

I suspect the upper fermenting gut is a root cause of many diseases and this is biologically plausible since most, if not all, have an infectious driver (see our book *The Infection Game*). Stomach cancer incidence has fallen as we diagnose and treat *H pylori*, but oesophageal cancer is the fastest rising cancer in Westerners.

In this regard, and as an aside, I have dealt with three cases of 'Barrett's oesophagus' by addressing upper gut fermentation. Barrett's is a pre-malignant lesion diagnosed by endoscopy (the camera down the throat). I treated all three patients with a combination of the PK diet and vitamin C to bowel tolerance (explained in Appendix 5). In all three cases, symptoms of reflux and indigestion disappeared quickly and follow-up endoscopy was much improved in one case and normal in the other two. One patient told me that his consultant said it was not possible for these interventions to afford a cure and that the original

---

*Abnormal fermentations in the upper gut are better recognised by vets. Cattle overfed on cereals may ferment these to D-lactic acid. D-lactic acidosis clinically looks like BSE and, indeed, 20% of cattle diagnosed clinically with BSE test negative for such – it is likely these beasts have D-lactic acidosis (and yes, we are still seeing new cases of BSE! Gosh – I could write another book on that subject). Horses allowed to eat too much sweet spring grass risk upper gut fermentation by a microbe that produces a toxin – this drives the devastatingly painful inflammation in the feet called laminitis.

diagnosis of Barrett's must have been incorrect.[†]

However, the most important feature for our Knackered Ape is that the fermenting gut drains us of energy for at least two reasons:

- the liver uses up energy and raw materials to deal with the toxic products of such a fermenting gut, and

- some of these toxins spill over into the bloodstream, resulting in foggy brain and malaise – ask anyone with a hangover.

The foggy brain

Listening to the exact words that patients use to describe how they feel affords vital clinical clues. So many tell me they feel poisoned and that often points to a fermenting gut issue.

Work by the Japanese researcher Nishihara[3] suggests that where there is a fermenting gut there is a fermenting brain. This ties in with recent research that firmly links the gut microbiome to brain pathology. Perhaps neurotransmitters in the brain are fermented to LSD and amphetamine-like substances? This may be the pathological basis of psychosis and explain the clinical triumphs of consultant psychiatrists Carl Pfeiffer and Abram Hoffer who successfully treated manic depression and schizophrenia with ketogenic diets.

By this stage you may be asking, 'So, what can I eat?' The answer is, as you will have gleaned in this chapter, the paleo-ketogenic (PK) diet. This is explained in Appendix 1 (page 140) and in much greater detail in our book *The PK Cookbook*.

[†]**Note from Craig:** Maybe the consultant is 'addicted' to Modern Western Practice and is therefore in denial, addiction and denial going hand in hand...

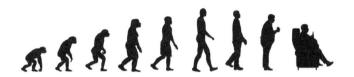

CHAPTER
7

ENERGY DELIVERY:

THE MITOCHONDRIAL ENGINE

Mitochondria are the common powerhouse for all multi-cellular eukaryotic organisms, from peanuts and pineapples to porcupines and professors. (For the biologists, prokaryotes – bacteria and 'archaea' – do not have mitochondria, but all eukaryotes do). I learned this at school and again at medical school. Indeed, mitochondria were central to our biochemistry curriculum. This was a subject mugged up the night before the exam – with the assistance of coffee, chocolate and fear of failure* – and forgotten as quickly because it apparently had no clinical application. It took me 10 years of clinical medicine before waking with a eureka moment. Those patients with chronic

---

*Note from Craig: Fear of failure can be a very strong driver. In the year above me at college, one chap had written the number 2 on large pieces of paper all over his study room walls. This was so that every time he looked up from his notes, he saw '2' and believed this was what he would be awarded (i.e. a 'Second' rather than a 'First') if he kept on looking at the wall rather than studying! In those days, Oxford University only awarded Firsts, Seconds, Thirds (and at one time Fourths too). Consequently, the vast majority of students were awarded a Second, making it almost meaningless. The Second class was divided into the familiar 2:1 and 2:2 in the early 1980s.

fatigue syndrome with whom I had been struggling... perhaps they had a mitochondrial problem?

How would I know whether my patients had a mitochondrial problem or not? I now realise how fortunate I was to be working with Dr John McLaren Howard. If anyone should win the Nobel Prize for Biochemistry it is John. Towards the end of the 1990s I felt brave enough to put to him the question of fatigue and how to measure mitochondrial function or, more accurately, dysfunction. Remember that John was not only brilliant but well established in his field compared with a minnow like myself. I felt it was like asking God for a miracle. At that time, I did not realise that his brilliance was matched by infinite kindness and generosity. Whilst I could ask the easy question – is it possible that fatigue could be partly explained by mitochondrial engine failure – it was up to John to develop a test so that we could evaluate this hypothesis and put into action its results.

A test for mitochondrial function

The role of mitochondria as central to Life is well accepted by evolutionary biologists, biochemists, anthropologists and other such experts. So why is it that mitochondria are nowhere to be seen in the medical world? Despite mitochondria making up 25% of the heart, even today they do not feature in cardiology. Despite the brain, weight for weight, requiring 10 times more energy than the rest of the body, mitochondria go without mention in neurological textbooks. The liver is rich in mitochondria to power the multiplicity of complex tasks it performs, but again, energy delivery mechanisms seem not to be a part of the hepatologist's differential diagnosis.

Now that I see human disease from the energy perspective, I cannot find a major pathology in which mitochondria are not involved. This is not surprising. Think of the complexity of modern human existence

– switch off the energy and everything fails. The body is the same. It is really quite astonishing that, despite the fabulous science, we still, today in 2021, have seen only one test that can measure mitochondrial function for clinical purposes.

As an analogy, imagine what would happen to modern Western society, if suddenly we lost our power generators (car engines, boilers, cookers, electricity generators)? Now substitute 'human body' for 'modern Western society' and 'mitochondrial produced energy' for 'power generators'.

By 2005, John had developed a test for mitochondrial function by adapting one already widely used in research laboratories to measure ATP – the energy molecule. If you wish to find out much more about ATP, read our book *Diagnosis and Treatment of Chronic Fatigue Syndrome and Mylagic Encephalitis – it's mitochondria not hypochondria*. Like any internal combustion engine, mitochondria take fuel (in the form of acetate groups) and burn it in the presence of oxygen to produce energy (in the form of the energy molecule ATP). There is some fascinating (albeit nasty when it has to be committed to memory for 24 hours) biochemistry to explain how this happens. However, all we need to know for clinical purposes is that ATP is the energy molecule. Think of it as money. With such we can purchase any job in the body, from contracting a muscle to conducting a nerve impulse and building new liver cells. It is as ancient and essential a molecule as DNA.

The brilliance of John's test was that it looked directly at the function of mitochondria – how good they were at making ATP, how efficiently this was moved from inside the mitochondria to the cell where it was needed for all energy requiring jobs, how efficiently and appropriately energy was released and, finally, how efficiently ADP (the spent molecule) was recycled back into mitochondria.

Through following and measuring ATP in its cycle, John could see where events were going slow. This has been so important in my treatment of patients with CFS and ME because it clearly shows that these people have a physical reason for their fatigue. Indeed, we could measure this objectively with a mitochondrial energy score. The first scientific paper authored by John McLaren Howard, Dr Norman Booth of Mansfield College Oxford and me showed that the sufferers of CFS with the worst fatigue had the lowest mitochondrial energy score and vice versa. However, more importantly, John's test showed up many of the reasons why mitochondria were going slow and this had very clear implications for management and treatment.[1]

We published a second paper in 2012[2] and a third in 2013 – a 'clinical audit'.[3] We could not get ethical committee approval or financial backing for a controlled study, and so this is why the follow-up study was in the form of an audit of 39 patients who underwent repeat tests. Despite this being a less than perfect study, the statistics were very powerful. All of those who underwent the necessary regimes improved their mitochondrial energy score. This showed that the biochemical lesions responded reliably well to the interventions as detailed below. To further reinforce the statistics, there were four patients who did not do the interventions and they all worsened their score.

Since that initial study I have done a further 1036 mitochondrial function tests (as at April 2020) and the clinical experience from those reinforces the findings from the clinical audit. As a result, I can treat patients with mitochondrial dysfunction even if they cannot access mitochondrial function tests, knowing that there should be a good response. The common biochemical lesions/problems that I see, why they occur and what we have to do to correct them are detailed next.

Table 7.1: Why mitochondria go slow and what to do about it

Mitochondria go slow because:	Car engines go slow because:	How to diagnose...	...and treat
They do not have the optimum fuel running...	You have put petrol into your diesel engine...	From the diet	PK diet
at the optimum rate	...and alternately starved the engine and/or flooded it	Ditto – wobbly blood sugar levels of metabolic syndrome	PK diet
They lack acetyl-L-carnitine which transports the acetate fuel from the body of the cell into mitochondria	The fuel pipe to the engine is narrowed	Blood tests for levels of acetyl-L-carnitine	Eat meat and/or supplement with up to 2 grams daily acetyl-L-carnitine
They lack oxygen to burn fuel where:	The air intake is narrowed		
• there is anaemia or poor circulation		Blood test for anaemia	Find the cause of the anaemia
• there is severe obstructive airways disease		Clinically obvious!	Find the cause
• there is poor blood supply		Low blood pressure and/or symptoms of poor circulation	Find the cause
They lack vitamin B3 (niacin) and/or magnesium	The fuel cannot be ignited	Blood test for NADH	Niacinamide 1500 mg daily
		Blood test for red cell magnesium	Magnesium 300 mg daily. Vitamin D 10,000 iu daily

Table 7.1: Why mitochondria go slow and what to do about it (cont.)

Mitochondria go slow because:	Car engines go slow because:	How to diagnose...	...and treat
They lack co-enzyme Q10	There is no oil to reduce friction	Blood tests for coQ10	CoQ10 100-200 mg daily
They have been blocked by • a toxin or poison such as a heavy metal, pesticide or volatile organic compound (VOC)...	You have thrown a handful of sand into the workings, clogged it up in unpredictable ways, increased friction and accelerated ageing	Tests of toxicity – see our book *Ecological Medicine*	Detox regimes work reliably well – see Chapter 12, The bare necessities
• or immunoproteins stuck onto mitochondrial membranes	Ditto	Look for a chronic infection – see our book *The Infection Game*. Suspect this if blood tests show inflammation – see Chapter 15, Getting your act together	Improve the immune defences. Use antimicrobials. Read *The Infection Game*
The control mechanisms are faulty	The accelerator pedal and gear box do not work	Read on for thyroid and adrenal problems	Take thyroid and adrenal glandulars

Why mitochondria go slow

Mitochondria go slow because they do not have the optimum fuel, at the optimum rate; they lack acetyl L carnitine for transporting fuel and oxygen for burning fuel; they lack key vitamins and minerals; they have been blocked by a toxin or immunoproteins; or their control mechanism is faulty. In Table 7.1 I explain each of these problems using the car analogy of earlier chapters and summarise how to diagnose and treat them.

Mitochondria are responsible for the ageing process – how to look after them

This is a great reason for us all to know about mitochondria. If mitochondria run very slowly then a critical moment arises when the cell does not have sufficient energy to run itself, let alone contribute to the collective needs of the whole body. The only hope for the survival of the whole is for that cell to commit suicide. Ageing is characterised by a loss of cells, which is particularly noticeable in muscles, and this is accelerated when energy delivery mechanisms go slow. Indeed, declining muscle mass is a good predictor of longevity, or rather, lack of it.

What this means is that if you look after your mitochondria you have a much better chance of living well to a great age and staying free of disease. So, this begs the question, what is the very least we have to do to achieve such, without having to go to the bother of expensive tests? My view is that, with increasing age and in order of importance, we must take the steps listed in Table 7.2.

Table 7.2: How to look after your mitochondria

What to consider	How to optimise mitochondrial function
Fuel	PK diet
Acetyl-L-carnitine	Having sufficient should not be a problem for meat-eaters (meat is a rich source of carnitine) who are following a PK diet (you need an acid stomach to digest protein) Vegetarians should take acetyl-L-carnitine 500 mg daily Anyone on acid-blocking drugs should do the same
Co-enzyme Q10	100 mg daily is sufficient for most; take this with a fatty meal to enhance absorption With any pathology take 200 mg
Niacinamide	1500 mg daily With any pathology, from psychosis to heart disease, double the dose

Table 7.2: How to look after your mitochondria (cont.)

What to consider	How to optimise mitochondrial function
D-ribose	Essential with any pathology Take 5-15 g daily but this must be part of the carbohydrate count of the PK diet (see Appendix 5)
Detox regime to get rid of toxic metals	Take a good multi-mineral, such as Sunshine salt, and combine with glutathione 250 mg Test for departing toxic metals by measuring urine elements following a dose of the chelating agent DMSA, 15 mg per kg body weight; this test is available through https://naturalhealthworldwide.com/lab-tests/
Detox regime to get rid of pesticides and VOCs	Once a week get very hot then wash sweat off in a bath or shower. If you are well enough to exercise then that is ideal, but sauna, far infrared sauna or a hot bath with Epsom salts are good too; these regimes are of proven benefit
Match energy demand to energy delivery	Read on – this is a thyroid and adrenal issue (see Chapter 8)
Enable service and repair	Read on – this is why sleep is so vital (see Chapter 9)
Work to increase numbers of mitochondria	Use it or lose it – • physical exercise produces lactic acid, and this stimulates the development of more mitochondria. • mental exercises such as crosswords, learning a new language or playing an instrument improve brain function. Thyroid hormones also determine the number of mitochondria (they give us a bigger engine)

As Eleanor Roosevelt said: *It takes as much energy to wish as it does to plan.* So, rather than just wishing you felt more energetic, you might as well plan to be more energetic, following the advice in both this chapter and the previous one. Then, when you have done the planning, just do it!

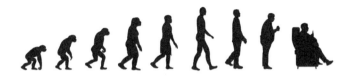

CHAPTER
8

MATCHING ENERGY GENERATION TO ENERGY DEMANDS

THE THYROID ACCELERATOR PEDAL AND THE ADRENAL GEAR BOX

The close matching of energy demands to delivery is of fundamental survival value. When a sabre-toothed tiger jumps out on primitive me, I need to put in an Olympic-performance sprint and that requires maximal energy delivery.*

Conversely, if I am resting up in a warm nest then I can reduce energy delivery commensurate with such. This balancing all happens courtesy of the adrenal and thyroid glands. Broadly speaking, the

*Note from Craig: Technically Sarah doesn't need to run faster than the sabre-toothed tiger; she only needs to run faster than the chap standing next to her – it's called Survival of the Fittest! Knowing Sarah as I do though, she'd probably start running, see that her fellow human was about to become sabre-toothed tiger supper, and then charge back and throttle said tiger.

thyroid gland base-loads to establish the basal metabolic rate and the adrenals fine tune. For a 'second to minute' response we have adrenalin which may be followed by a 'minute to hourly' response determined by cortisol. Hibernating bears have low levels of thyroid hormone; we see levels of thyroid hormones in humans increase in the summer. This makes perfect evolutionary sense.

Doctors have long failed to grasp the vital therapeutic significance of diet, micronutrients and mitochondria. This poor record continues with respect to thyroid and adrenal function. Whilst absolute failures are diagnosed and treated, partial failures are not. There is a large grey area between 100% and zero function which grows with age and fatigue but goes unrecognised by endocrinologists. Conventional blood tests for thyroid and adrenal function are blunt tools, commonly misinterpreted. Doctors use tests as an excuse to dismiss patients despite their clinical symptoms and so the need to treat is missed. Essentially, if the test results lie within population reference ranges, then the thinking stops. The clinical picture is ignored. The fatigued patient is dismissed.

Hypothyroidism is already common (about 10% of Westerners have underactive thyroid) and is underdiagnosed (less than 2% receive treatment). Dr Kenneth Blanchard, consultant endocrinologist, estimates that up to 40% of American women are hypothyroid and would benefit from thyroid hormones. (For much more detail see our book *Ecological Medicine*.) It is my experience that, of the naive patients who consult me complaining of fatigue, all have metabolic syndrome, most have a thyroid issue, many have an adrenal problem and the severely fatigued also have mitochondrial failure.

Do I have thyroid or adrenal hypofunction as a cause of my fatigue?

Suspect hypothyroidism if you continue to suffer from many of the symptoms detailed in Chapter 3 *despite* eating a PK diet *and* taking a basic package of micronutrients *and* being seen by a doctor who has told you that pathology has been excluded and nothing more can be done.

What can I do to fix this?

The first thing is to measure levels of the hormones thyroid-stimulating hormone (TSH), free thyroxin (T4) and free T3 in the blood just to make quite sure that the converse is not true (i.e. rule out you are not *hyper*thyroid, with an over-active gland). One would think the clinical pictures were completely different, but sometimes the thyrotoxic patient (patient with too much thyroxin) presents with fatigue. This blood test can be easily done on a DIY finger-drop sample of blood and sent to a laboratory (see https://naturalhealthworldwide.com/ for labs that offer this test).

For the fine-tuning of our engine we have to rely on the clinical picture. This can be done through measuring core temperature, pulse rate and blood pressure together with the 'how do you feel' test.

If the above suggest that there is biochemical and clinical scope for a clinical trial of a treatment, we can hypothesise that there is hypothyroidism. We then put that hypothesis to the test and go ahead with a trial. Remember, all diagnosis is retrospective. If the symptoms of Chapter 3 are ameliorated and the core temperatures, pulse and blood pressure normalise, then the hypothesis is confirmed and the diagnosis made. That is to say if the treatment works, then the diagnosis follows.

This combined problem of thyroid and adrenal grey areas is so common, with patients being dismissed by doctors, that already we have, I estimate, hundreds of thousands of sufferers who have taken matters into their own hands and elected to treat themselves. I have seen many such and always been impressed by their knowledge and diagnostic acumen. Between us all, a safe and effective framework for recovery has evolved.

The 'tools of the trade': glandulars

Glandulars make effective therapy possible. For thyroid disease we can use thyroid glandulars, for adrenal disease, adrenal glandulars. These are simply dried thyroid and adrenal glands from pigs or cows. But how to get the dose right?

The 'rules of the game': glandulars

You should start glandulars and keep on increasing the dose until:

- Your average core temperature is 37°C, but do not start or increase doses if this is above 37°C (see table 8.1)

- Your average daily wobble in temperature readings is less than 0.5°C.

You should not start or increase doses of glandulars if:

- Your resting pulse rate is above 85 bpm; you must bring this down by the PK diet and previous interventions (including addressing mitochondrial function) before starting or increasing doses of glandulars

- Your resting blood pressure is above 120/80 mm Hg; you must bring this down by the PK diet and previous interventions (including addressing mitochondrial function) before starting or increasing doses of glandulars.

There is more detail in Table 8.1.

Table 8.1: The dos and don'ts of using glandulars effectively

What	Why
You must be on a PK diet	With metabolic syndrome we see wobbly blood sugar levels. As blood sugar falls, adrenalin is released. Adrenalin plus glandulars may give all the symptoms of too much adrenalin – this is very uncomfortable and the commonest reason for intolerance of glandulars
Your average core temperature must be below 37ºC. This is a reflection of thyroid function	Core temperature is a good measure of one's combined energy delivery mechanisms – i.e. the PK fuel in the tank, the mitochondrial engine, the thyroid accelerator pedal and the adrenal gear box. If core temperature is too high, then energy delivery is too fast. This occurs naturally when one runs a fever to deal with infection
The degree of wobble (the difference between the lowest temperature of the day and the highest) should be less that 0.5 of a degree C. This is a reflection of adrenal function	The adrenal gland matches energy delivery to demand on a second to minute to hours basis. Any mismatch is a waste of energy. That means there is less energy to spend on life
Your resting pulse rate must be below 85 bpm (beats per minute) (As you improve all energy delivery mechanisms, the pulse rate will come down to 70-75 bpm – this is because the heart can beat with greater power and so can run more slowly)	It is the thyroid gland that determines resting pulse rate. However, for patients who are severely fatigued, the resting pulse may be high – this is because when mitochondrial function is so poor the heart does not have the energy to beat powerfully so the only way it can increase output for basal metabolism is to beat faster. An extreme example of this is postural orthostatic tachycardia syndrome characterised by very low blood pressure that drops further on standing whilst the pulse races to compensate for the low cardiac output
Your resting blood pressure must be below 120/80 mm Hg	It is a feature of the severely fatigued patient that they have low blood pressure for the above reasons. High blood pressure is typical of metabolic syndrome (a further reason to go PK)

Table 8.1: The dos and don'ts of using glandulars effectively (cont.)

What	Why
You are not functioning at your full potential because of fatigue	Keep a diary of which symptoms and how severe; it is easy to forget Note from Craig: From my experience, sometimes I forgot as a kind of internal coping mechanism, a way of surviving, almost a self-inflicted denial of how bad things were. My wife, Penny, tells me the same is true of childbirth

What, when and how much?

These dose suggestions are made with respect to the commercially available products, Adrenavive II and III, and Metavive I and II. Other glandulars contain different amounts of active ingredients and so doses will need to be adjusted accordingly.

- Start with 40 mg of thyroid glandular and increase in 40 mg increments every two weeks according to average core temperatures and the check list above.

- Start with 150 mg of adrenal cortex glandular and increase in 150 mg increments every week according to the range (or wobble) of core temperature and the check list above. If despite getting to 900-1200 mg of adrenal cortex glandular, the core temperature is still wobbling, then this may point to your body's attempt to run a fever to get rid of a chronic infection. See our book *The Infection Game* for much more detail.

- Most people need daily doses of 900-1200 mg of thyroid glandular. For many, the last 15 mg seems to make the world of difference.

- Most need 300-900 mg of adrenal cortex glandular to feel well.

- Both should be taken in two doses, half on rising, half at midday.

- Bigger people need a higher dose than little people.

- Many people vary the dose a little from day to day to deal with demand.

- As we age the prevalence of hypothyroidism and poor adrenal function increases.

What are the long-term risks of glandulars?

The key point to remember is that the dose is critical. Without thyroid and adrenal hormones, we die. With inadequate amounts we risk disease and premature death – poor quality and quantity of life.

The two commonest complications cited of mild over-dosing are atrial fibrillation (irregular and often rapid heart rate) and osteoporosis. So, should we be worried about this? The key point here is that both these conditions are multifactorial and, by paying attention to all factors, the risk of any such complication is mitigated.

a) **Atrial fibrillation**. There are two major risk factors for this. Firstly, metabolic syndrome, which is completely reversible with a PK diet. The second common cause is heavy metal toxicity. This is mitigated by taking the basic package of nutritional supplements, particularly friendly minerals, vitamin C and glutathione. If there is any history of toxic metal exposure, then this can be easily measured on a urine sample following DMSA as explained on my website – www.drmyhill.co.uk/wiki/Toxic_elements_in_urine_following_DMSA

b) **Osteoporosis**. Again, the major risk factor for this is metabolic syndrome. This is followed by lack of exercise; of course, correcting thyroid and adrenal function gives the patient the energy to do such. Adrenal hormones, especially DHEA, protect against osteoporosis. Should there be any concern, then one can safely measure bone density using heel ultrasound (no radiation, minimal cost – see http://bonematters.org/) and treatment with natural strontium 250 mg daily is of proven effectiveness and very safe. Do not use the synthetic strontium ranelate which is formulated with aspartame.

Why are thyroid and adrenal disorders so common?

Adrenal fatigue I suspect is also part of metabolic syndrome. Wobbly blood sugar levels are stressful to the body. Sugar is a very damaging molecule – it is sticky and that results in sticky blood and damage to the lining of arteries. Insulin is employed to control high blood sugar so down come the levels. Suddenly there may be insufficient to fuel the sugar-adapted mitochondria and energy delivery starts to shut down. Panic! Release the instant panic hormone adrenalin, which is followed by cortisol, DHEA and others. Metabolic syndrome is characterised by spiking adrenal hormones so, not surprisingly, the adrenal gland gets fatigued. This increases its need for raw materials, especially vitamin C, and this is the commonest micronutrient deficiency in humans.

The causes of thyroid dysfunction are listed in Table 8.2.

So, where are we now? We have learned why things have gone wrong. We have learned how to generate energy – diet and mitochondria. We have just learned how to match energy supply with energy demand, thereby avoiding wasting energy. Now it is time to talk of sleep. Shakespeare got it right when he wrote in Henry IV: '*O sleep! O gentle sleep! Nature's soft nurse.*' (From *Henry IV Part II*, Act III Scene 1, '*Enter the King in his nightgown, with a page*'.) Let's investigate this nurse… we need her on side.

Table 8.2: The causes of thyroid dysfunction

Reasons for poor thyroid function	Why?	How to mitigate
There is no kick from the pituitary gland – this is called 'secondary hypothyroidism'	This is the commonest form of hypothyroidism in my CFS patients. I suspect poisoning by chemicals, especially organophosphates (glyphosate – Roundup – is among these) and lack of vitamin B12 are important players	Avoid chemical exposure – try to eat organic Heating regimes to get rid of toxins
The thyroid gland lacks iodine to make thyroid hormones	Iodine deficiency is pandemic	Take iodine 1 mg daily
The thyroid has been poisoned by:		
• fluoride	...from fluoridated water, toothpaste and/or dental treatments	Avoid fluoride
• and/or bromide	...from polybrominated biphenyls (PBBs) used as fire retardants in soft furnishings	Avoid Heating regimes to get rid of bromides
• toxic metals: mercury, lead, cadmium and aluminium	These heavy metals bio-accumulate so past exposures are always significant: Mercury from dental amalgam, fish, vaccinations Lead from old water pipes, old paints Cadmium from cigarette smoke, water Aluminium from deodorants, vaccinations, cooking utensils	Avoid Take minerals, vitamin C and glutathione to help excrete these
• mycotoxins	...from water-damaged buildings and/or low-grade infection, most often chronic sinusitis	Avoid Measure urinary mycotoxins (see page 186)

Table 8.2: The causes of thyroid dysfunction (cont.)

Reasons for poor thyroid function	Why?	How to mitigate
The thyroid has been destroyed by autoimmunity	Autoimmune conditions now affect 20% of Westerners	The main risk factors for autoimmunity are vaccination, vitamin D deficiency and dairy products. Once the thyroid has been destroyed it cannot grow back; replacement therapy will be needed for life
The thyroid has been destroyed by infection	Infection may be viral, bacterial or fungal	Once the thyroid has been destroyed it cannot grow back; replacement therapy will be needed for life
Deficiency of selenium, zinc and/ or iron	These minerals are necessary to allow the conversion of inactive T4 to active T3	Take daily multi-mineral such as Sunshine salt
Thyroid hormone receptor resistance (THRR)	The thyroid hormones are present, but the receptors are blocked; this may result in high levels of reverse T3 or toxic chemicals and heavy metals. I suspect there is an element of THRR as part of metabolic syndrome	Avoid toxic chemicals and heavy metals Mitigate toxic chemicals and heavy metals as above PK diet Measure reverse T3 – a high rT3 is one cause of THRR
A cocktail of some or all the above	...and this is usually the case!	Do your best with all the above Supplement with thyroid glandulars

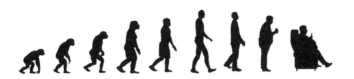

CHAPTER
9

SLEEP

Sleep is the golden chain that ties health and our bodies together.
Thomas Dekker (c.1572 – 1632)

Why we sleep

All living creatures have times in their cycle when they shut down their metabolic activity for healing and repair to take place. Without such they die. Dolphins, who must constantly swim, achieve such by shutting down one side of their brains at a time. Swifts, who can be airborne for 10 months, have learned to sleep on the wing. During the 'flu epidemic after the First World War, a few sufferers developed neurological damage in which they lost the ability to sleep. All were dead within two weeks – this was the first solid evidence that sleep is an absolute essential for life. The condition familial fatal insomnia is characterised by increasing insomnia, hallucinations, dementia and death.

Chronic lack of sleep kills us in road traffic accidents, with a greater facility than alcohol. It also drives diabetes, heart disease, cancer and dementia. Sleep deprivation is a torture – 16th century Scottish 'witches' were deprived of sleep until they hallucinated and so 'confessed'. It was chronic sleep deprivation which determined that I would not be pursuing a junior hospital doctor career. Indeed, there is no disease process that is not worsened by lack of sleep. It really is a risk factor for all disease. Quantity and quality of sleep are non-negotiable.

Embrace '*Nature's soft nurse*'.

Sleep is essential but why is that? The answer is energy and use. No energy-generating system is perfect. Energy, employed by all living creatures, is generated when sunshine interacts with water; in the process, free radicals (unstable chemicals) are produced, and these create damage. So do wear and tear. During sleep we heal and repair. If there is insufficient sleep, then the cell damage exceeds healing and repair and our health gradually ratchets downhill.

Happily, the body has a symptom which tells us how much sleep we need. It is called sleepiness and is characterised by yawning – ignore it at your peril.

During sleep, the glymphatics, the rubbish disposal systems of the brain, open up to allow cleaning, healing and repair. An example of such rubbish is amyloid, the pathological protein of Alzheimer's disease. This is cleared from the brain during sleep. If sleep is lacking, then amyloid builds up in the brain. Lack of sleep is a major risk factor for dementia.

Without a good night's sleep on a regular basis, all other interventions are to no avail. There are at least three aspects to pay attention to: the quantity of sleep, when to sleep (circadian rhythm) and the quality of sleep.

The quantity of sleep

Modern Western man is chronically sleep deprived. He averages 7.5 hours of sleep when the biological average requirement is nearer 9 hours, perhaps a bit more in winter, less in summer. To show how critical this balance is, imagine dividing the day into 12 hours of activity and 12 hours of rest. One extra hour of damaging activity (13 hours) means the loss of one hour of rest and healing sleep (11 hours). As you can see, the difference is two hours. It is vital to observe a regular bedtime and to be able to wake naturally, without an alarm clock, feeling refreshed.

When to sleep (circadian rhythm*)

Humans evolved to sleep when it is dark and to be awake when it is light. Sleep is a form of hibernation when the body shuts down in order to repair damage done through use, to conserve energy and to hide from predators. The normal sleep pattern that evolved in hot climates is to sleep, keep warm and conserve energy during the cold nights and then sleep again in the afternoons when it is too hot to work and to hide away from the midday sun. As humans migrated away from the Equator, the sleep pattern had to change with the seasons and as the lengths of the days changed. In winter we need to shut down to conserve energy – this means more sleep. Mild fatigue and depression in winter prevent us from spending energy unnecessarily. Conversely,

Historical note: Franz Halberg (5 July 1919 – 9 June 2013) coined the word 'circadian' in 1959 by combining two Latin words – '*circa*' (about) and '*diem*', accusative singular of '*dies*' (day). Halberg was a maverick, working seven days a week, right up to his death, who spoke of the 'quicksand of clinical trials on groups' and that 'These [clinical trials] ignore individual differences and hence the individual's needs.'

in the summer we need to expend large amounts of energy to harvest the summer bounties and accumulate reserves to carry us through the winter; we naturally need less sleep, can work longer hours and have more energy. But the need for a rest (if not a sleep) in the middle of the day is still there. Therefore, it is no surprise that young children, the elderly and people who become ill often have an extra sleep in the afternoon and for these people that is totally desirable. Others have learned to 'power nap', as it is called, during the day and this allows them to feel more energetic later. If you can do it then this is an excellent habit to get into – it can be learned. The average daily sleep requirement is nine hours, ideally taken between 9.30 pm and 6.30 am – that is, during the hours of darkness – but allow for more in the winter and less in the summer. An hour of sleep before midnight is worth two after; this is because human growth hormone is produced during the hours of sleep before midnight.

An hour of sleep before midnight is worth two after
Well known saying… and Mother was right, again!

Early to bed and early to rise, makes a man healthy, wealthy and wise.
Benjamin Franklin[†] (17 January 1706 – 17 April 1790)

The symptoms of jet lag are a powerful illustration of the existence

[†]**Historical note:** We do have Franklin to thank for bringing this well-known phrase into common usage (my mother said this to me an awful lot during my teenage years, always with a strong emphasis on the 'wise' – Craig) but there are earlier versions, showing that indeed this wisdom has been known for hundreds of years. In *The Boke of Saint Albans*, printed in 1486, we have: '*As the olde englysshe prouerbe sayth in this wyse. Who soo woll ryse erly shall be holy helthy & zely*'. The Middle English word 'zely' had numerous meanings in 1486 but foremost were 'auspicious' or 'fortunate'. So 'holy helthy & zely' meant 'wise, healthy and fortunate'. *The Boke of Saint Albans* contains advice on hawking, hunting and heraldry with a chapter on fishing added in 1496.[2]

of a circadian rhythm. The rhythm starts with light which shines on the skin (interestingly not necessarily through the eyes) and switches off melatonin production. As darkness ensues, melatonin is produced to create the hormonal environment for sleep. Melatonin stimulates the pituitary gland to produce thyroid stimulating hormone (TSH) and this peaks at midnight. The thyroid is stimulated to produce T4 (thyroxin) which spikes at 4 am. This is converted to the active thyroid hormone T3 which spikes at 5 am. T3 kicks the adrenals into life and the rising levels of adrenalin, cortisol and DHEA wakes us up at 6-7 am.

My guess is that it is the varying levels of all these hormones through the night that determine the proportion of non-REM to REM sleep (see below) and this too is critical for good health. Good thyroid and adrenal function is essential for good quality sleep. A further likely mechanism for sleep is the effect on core temperature. Indeed, there is a very clear relationship between onset of sleep and falling core temperature, and this is achieved by increasing blood flow to the skin, so heat is lost.

The quality of sleep

There are two recognisable types of sleep, called rapid eye movement (REM) sleep and non-REM sleep. We see a cycle of these every 90 minutes. Non-REM sleep comes first and during this time we sort through the experiences of the day and store the important ones, essential to survival, as memory. We then slip into REM sleep during which we dream, and problem solve. All sorts of odd connections are made. We start the night with a high proportion of non-REM to REM sleep and finish the night with proportionately more REM sleep. As I have said, I suspect the relative proportions are determined by the changing levels of the hormones melatonin, T3 and T4 and adrenal hormones which occur through the sleep cycle. It is easy to see how both sorts of sleep confer survival advantage. We do not want to clog up the brain with useless memories and we need to make lots of bizarre connections for problem solving.

An appreciation of the importance of sleep is not new. For non-REM sleep and its function of sorting and storing important memories, we have the following from *A Study in Scarlet* by Sir Arthur Conan Doyle[‡]. Sherlock Holmes is speaking:

> *I consider that a man's brain originally is like a little empty attic, and you have to stock it with such furniture as you choose. A fool takes in all the lumber of every sort that he comes across, so that the knowledge which might be useful to him gets crowded out, or at best is jumbled up with a lot of other things, so that he has a difficulty in laying his hands upon it. Now the skilful workman is very careful indeed as to what he takes into his brain-attic. He will have nothing but the tools which may help him in doing his work, but of these he has a large assortment, and all in the most perfect order. It is a mistake to think that that little room has elastic walls and can distend to any extent. Depend upon it there comes a time when for every addition of knowledge, you forget something that you knew before. It is of the highest importance, therefore, not to have useless facts elbowing out the useful ones.*

[‡]**Footnote:** Sir Arthur Conan Doyle (22 May 1859 – 7 July 1930) was buried in 1930 and again in 1955. He was not a Christian, considering himself a 'Spiritualist' and so he was first buried on 11 July 1930 in Windlesham rose garden. His body was later reinterred together with his wife's in Minstead churchyard in the New Forest, Hampshire.

For REM sleep we have the recommendation of Linus Pauling (28 February 1901 – 19 August 1994, and a major researcher into vitamin C): '*The key to having good ideas is to get lots of ideas and throw out the bad ones.*'

We end with more from Thomas Dekker and, as Craig's wife, Penny, used to sing to their children every night:

> *Golden slumbers kiss your eyes,*
> *Smiles awake you when you rise;*
> *Sleep, pretty wantons, do not cry*
> *And I will sing a lullaby,*
> *Rock them, rock them, lullaby.*
> *Care is heavy, therefore sleep you,*
> *You are care, and care must keep you;*
> *Sleep, pretty wantons, do not cry,*
> *And I will sing a lullaby,*
> *Rock them, rock them, lullaby.*

> *The Cradle Song,* by Thomas Dekker
> (c. 1572 – 25 August 1632)
> English dramatist and pamphleteer.

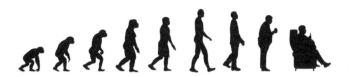

CHAPTER
10

OPTIMISING ENERGY EXPENDITURE THROUGH EXERCISE

THE BARE MINIMUM

Scene from Craig's pure mathematics class, 1980:

Mr Smith, Teacher – '*The best mathematicians are lazy*'
A N Other Student – '*But Sir, the best* people *are lazy*'
Craig – '*Oh, I can't be bothered with this discussion*'

Mr Smith and the student were both correct because all creatures are intrinsically lazy. This is an essential evolutionary survival tool for the business of energy conservation. Nature must carefully match energy expenditure with survival needs because energy wasted risks failure to survive the next famine, or fight infection. She gives us the bare minimum of bone structure, muscle and brain power to survive because anything more than that is energy wasted.

Exercise is eschewed by most Knackered Apes because it is hard work and painful. Worse, we do not exercise because we don't have to. Petrol, diesel and electricity see to that. At the same time, we know that physical fitness is an essential for good physical and mental health. Even Pooh Bear knew that; as he says: '*A bear however hard he tries, grows tubby without exercise*' (AA Milne, 1882 – 1956).

So, we have to ask our idle Naked Ape, what is the bare minimum that we can get away with? I do not see rabbits and foxes jogging round my hill every morning to keep fit – so how do they stay so well? Around once a week there is a predator-prey interaction when either the rabbit has to run for his life to prevent him becoming breakfast, or the fox has to run for his life to eat his breakfast. For both parties there would be a chase during which heart and muscles would be at maximum output. At the end of the chase, the survivor would have aching muscles and be gasping for breath. This is all that is necessary for fitness and this gives us the principles for the minimalist, modern, lazy Naked Ape (and yes, I can be one too).

- You just need to do enough to cause lactic acid burn but not cause any strain or injury - enough to make you puff and pant and get your heart rate up. The exercise has to be very slow but powerful – this prevents damage to muscles and joints. For the legs and heart, walk up a hill as fast as is possible. For the arms and core muscles, do press-ups. A rough rule of thumb for maximal heart rate is to subtract your age from 220. For me, aged 60, that is 160 beats per minute. (The mathematician in me immediately wonders what is maximal for the 219-year-old, or even the 221-year-old? – Craig.)

- It must be sufficiently powerful that the muscles being worked burn with lactic acid and weaken – that is to say, the exercise cannot be sustained any longer. What makes muscles fatigue is not lack of muscle filaments, but inability to supply energy to them.

- You may be tired at the end of the day, but you should feel completely recovered the next day. Poor recovery points to over-training. This is a feature of my CFS/ME patients and so they must pace activity very carefully until energy delivery mechanisms are restored

We need to do the 'just enough' amount of exercise – like Goldilocks:*

'This porridge is too hot!' she exclaimed.
So, she tasted the porridge from the second bowl.
'This porridge is too cold,' she said.
So, she tasted the last bowl of porridge.
'Ahhh, this porridge is just right,' she said
happily, and she ate it all up.

*Historical note: *Goldilocks and the Three Bears* (originally entitled *The Story of the Three Bears*) is a British 19th-century fairy tale, first recorded in narrative form by British writer and poet Robert Southey (1774 – 1843). There are at least three versions of this tale: the first tells of a grumpy old woman who enters the home of three bachelor bears whilst they are away. She sits in their chairs, eats some of their porridge, and sleeps in one of their beds. When the bears return and discover her, she wakes up, jumps out of the window and is never seen again. The second version replaced the old woman with a little girl named Goldilocks, and the third and most well-known version replaced the original bear trio with Papa Bear, Mama Bear and Baby Bear.

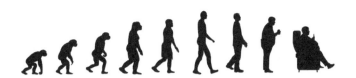

CHAPTER
11

FREE ENERGY

SOMETHING FOR NOTHING

At first reading, the title of this chapter sounds as though we have discovered some kind of perpetual motion machine. The dream of so many throughout the ages has been to create a machine that worked indefinitely without an energy source. Leonardo da Vinci knew that this was a futile quest when he said: '*Oh ye seekers after perpetual motion, how many vain chimeras have you pursued? Go and take your place with the alchemists.*' (1494).

We now know in more well-defined science – the laws of thermodynamics – why truly getting something for nothing is not possible. This is not what we are discussing here, however. This chapter represents a summary of Professor Gerald Pollack's book, *The Fourth Phase of Water*. Interested Naked and Knackered Apes are encouraged to buy and read it.

The fourth phase of water

Professor Gerald Pollack describes a fourth phase of water. We are all familiar with solid ice, liquid water and water vapour/steam. The fourth phase occurs when water molecules lie against a surface, such as a cell membrane, protein or ion. The slightly polar (magnet-like) water molecules organise themselves into layers of honeycomb hexagons which have remarkable properties. The structure is such that protons are squeezed out; consequently the honeycomb is negatively charged and the liquid water beyond is positively charged. Pollack calls this 'exclusion zone', or 'EZ', water. When this occurs in a cell and salts are present, there is a further separation of salts. Magnesium and potassium accumulate inside the cell and sodium and calcium outside. This occurs without any expenditure of energy from the cell. Indeed, this will happen with any semi-permeable membrane sphere. You do not get organised EZ water (for the physicists this is decreasing entropy) nor charge separation (like charging up a battery) for nothing – these processes require energy. So where is the energy coming from to allow EZ water to form? Well to answer that question, we have to think like Professor Gerald Pollack, who said: 'Discovery consists of seeing what everybody has seen and thinking what nobody has thought.'

EZ water creates a battery effect

We have known for years that partitioning of ions across cell membranes happens and explained this in terms of sodium/potassium   and calcium/magnesium ion pumps. Many other ion pumps have also been described. However, there is a big energy problem with all of this – if you tot up all the energy needed to maintain these ion pumps, it greatly exceeds the capacity of the cell to generate energy. For example, it has been calculated that the sodium pump alone would account for 30-35% of the cell's entire energy supply. Pollack himself recognised this as a problem. So, where does this energy for ion gradients come from?

EZ water drives circulation through capillaries

It has always been a mystery to me as to how blood circulates through the smallest of our blood vessels, namely capillaries. There is no pressure difference between the arterial and the venous ends since blood pressure is controlled by the pre-capillary arterioles. Worse, the bore of a capillary is about 5 microns and a red blood cell 8 microns – the red blood cells have to twist and distort to pass through. EZ water, however, explains this. EZ water lining capillaries is negatively charged, as is EZ water surrounding red cells. The electrical forces repel and push the red cells into a twisted shape. The liquid water between is positively charged, so this has a driving force from the arterial end (as blood is squeezed by declining blood vessel diameter) and a pulling force from the venous end (with expanding blood vessel diameter). Blood flows because it is driven by these localised electrical forces. Again, this process requires energy. Again, where does this come from?

EZ water increases elasticity, explains vesicles and enables ion pumps

Elastic tissue is comprised of long protein polymers surrounded by the EZ honeycomb water. If there is a divalent cation (positively charged ion with a valence* of 2) such as calcium, then this forms a bridge between the EZ honeycomb of adjacent polymers and pulls them together. However, if there is a monovalent cation (positively charged ion with a valence of 1) such as potassium, then this bridging does not happen and the honeycomb of polymers unzips and this causes stretching. So, calcium causes shrinkage and potassium causes stretching, meaning

*Valence is a measure of the combining power of the ion with other atoms when it forms compounds or molecules – the higher the valence, the higher the combining power.

that tiny changes in the concentrations of those two elements will flip these polymers from contraction (shrinkage) to stretching.

It is a similar mechanism that creates ion pumps. These protein polymers lie across cell membranes (they make up 50-80% of membranes) and flip from one form to another; in doing so they may flip molecules out and molecules in. Indeed, the one with which I am most familiar is translocator protein on mitochondrial membranes that flips ATP out of, and ADP back into, mitochondria for recycling.

This protein polymer shrinking explains *rigor mortis*. I could never understand why a corpse, which had no energy delivery mechanisms, would go stiff with muscle contraction and remain so for some hours. With death, calcium floods into cells and zips up the muscle fibres, sticking them together so that the muscle is unable to stretch. It is only decomposition that terminates *rigor mortis*. That explains why cold extends the time it lasts.

EZ water reduces friction between tissues

EZ honeycomb water lines all tissue surfaces and is electrically charged. As a result, there is no physical contact, other than water, between tissue layers. They slide over each other without friction, like a pair of repelling magnets, and so without pain. In joints like the knee, the synovial membrane is markedly negative. Between, the synovial fluid is markedly positive. All these repelling forces mean that there is no solid contact between the weight bearing surfaces of the joint despite many kilograms of pressure. What happens when the knee gets cold? The EZ honeycomb thins, charge separation lessens, there is more friction and possibly pain.

Free energy from background heat and radiation

Pollack found that EZ water would not form without background radiation. This is where the energy comes from to form EZ honeycombs. In practice this means that where you have any surface (a membrane, protein or charged ion), water and sunshine you have free energy. Sunshine (as ever) 'provides' the energy, in the form of background radiation. This is a great survival asset, and all Life takes advantage.

Pollack found that all wavelengths give us free energy, ultraviolet the least so, visible light moderately so but best is far infrared (FIR) light, particularly at a wavelength of 3000 nm (sunshine has all these wavelengths). What this means is that some, possibly much, of the energy necessary for an electrical impulse to run along nerves and muscles, for the release of neurotransmitters from vesicles, for muscular contraction and for capillary circulation, comes from outside the body – we absorb energy from the sun and use this for movement, communication, circulation and much more. This is free energy because we don't have to do anything to get it.

Mr Micawber (see page 16) would be ecstatic. It is as though he had found a purse that kept on being replenished with pennies as fast as he spent them – no more misery for him!

The group of animals knows as *Poikilotherms* are even more dependent on free energy to get started – lizards and snakes seek out sunshine to sunbathe and get going. As we humans age and energy delivery mechanisms decline, we all need more warming up to get going.

How do we feel when we are receiving free energy?

We feel well. We feel comfortable. We feel happy. Since free energy is so desirable, the brain gives us the symptoms necessary to harvest as much as is possible. So how do we feel in sunshine, heat and bright light? We feel well because we have energy. We all perceive this. I feel jolly when the sun is shining. I love to sunbathe. We all feel a bit depressed in the winter and get miserable in the cold. Who does not benefit from a winter holiday in the bright sunshine and warmth that ski-resorts give us?

My Patterdale terrier, Nancy, loves to stretch out in front of an open fire and stays there even when she's panting. So, do I! Stripey, the cat, loved to sunbathe. We love hot baths and saunas. Children in school perform better sitting next to a window. Modern office blocks eschew walls for windows and get more work out of their employees as a result.

How do heat and light make us feel well?

Heat, especially far infra-red (FIR) heat, improves capillary circulation and so areas of damage can heal and repair.

FIR increases the thickness of the EZ honeycomb water; this reduces friction between tissues and any associated symptom, so stiffness is improved. With age and pathology, many people report feeling 'stiff' in the morning and take a few minutes to warm up and move freely. Being stiff means more friction and so we need even more energy to move at all.

EZ water physically excludes molecules that do not 'fit' – since the EZ honeycomb thickens with heat; this may be the mechanism by which heating regimes reduce our load of xenobiotic chemicals (especially pesticides and volatile organic compounds) – they are physically squeezed out.

EZ water explains the elasticity of tissues – the electrical charge holds tissues like a stretched elastic band. About 40% of muscle power derives from such stored energy in elastic tissue, which then recharges during relaxation. This makes kangaroos, who rely on masses of elastic tissue, one of the most efficient movers over the ground. No EZ water and elasticity is impossible.

Other benefits of EZ water

Free energy from EZ water also explains:

- Athletes and 'second wind'. During exercise muscles generate heat in the form of FIR light and this further improves circulation, reduces friction, increases elasticity and energy delivery. I think this explains the phenomena of 'second wind' experienced by middle distance runners when, after an initial effort, running suddenly feels easier because heat improves EZ honeycombing and so we see more elasticity, better capillary circulation and less friction between tissue layers. A symptom of second wind is that skin temperature increases, again supporting the free heat explanation.

- Why people living in hot climates have mitochondria which run slower (and vice versa). Inuits have a BMR (basal metabolic rate) that is 16-18% higher than Europeans and Europeans have a BMR that is 5% higher than Africans. Glean free energy from the sun and you do not need to generate it yourself – this has great evolutionary survival value.

How do we harvest free energy?

Ignore risible Establishment advice to eschew sunshine. There is no evidence that ultraviolet causes the only dangerous skin cancer – namely, melanoma. There is also no evidence that sun-blockers protect against skin cancer. Get as much sunshine as you possibly can (without actually burning). Even if the sun is not shining, free energy is still pouring through the clouds.

If indoors, aim to position yourself as much as you can by windows and harvest the heat and light that pours through. Glass cuts out the ultraviolet rays but allows all others through. I am so lucky to be able to work in a sun-room. I know I can work longer hours and feel better in this bright light and FIR heat.

If you cannot work by a window, use full spectrum light bulbs, not narrow spectrum LEDs.

Room temperature for efficient work should be about 22°C (72°F). We can harvest energy from this, but not waste energy trying to cool off. If your comfortable room heat is more than this, then that suggests you have poor energy delivery mechanisms, and something must be done.

- Start with the PK diet.

- Aim for a regular hot bath, hot shower and/or traditional or FIR sauna to rebuild your EZ honeycombs. (Yes, I know this is a temporary fix but the effects persist for some hours afterwards.)

- Expose as much skin to light and heat so that clothing does not block energy absorption. Indeed, I wonder if this is part of the mechanism by which being over-weight is associated with poor energy. It is not just a power-weight ratio. Adipose tissue blocks the effect of direct heat and light on muscle and connective tissue so people with too much of it cannot benefit fully from free energy.

- Do not allow yourself to get cold – indeed, getting cold is such an uncomfortable feeling that we already take great measures to prevent it from happening. But putting an extra layer of clothing on is not as effective as increasing ambient temperature. That is why we all ignore Establishment advice to turn the heating down and put a jumper on.

- Aim FIR light on to any area of pain or friction (easy to use, cheap to buy).

- Finally, at night we shut down energy delivery mechanisms to allow sleep, healing and repair and so a cool bedroom affords better quality sleep. Although the official recommendation is 15.5-19.5°C (60-67°F), my view is that lower is better. If you need near to 19.5°C to be comfortable, that again points to poor energy delivery mechanisms.

Free energy and free fuel from fermenting fibre

Fibre is fermented by friendly microbes in the large bowel. That fermentation process generates heat and warms us up. It costs us nothing. Ruminants, such as horses and cows, ferment huge amounts of fibre – a cow's rumen contains up to 200 litres of ferment. This generates so much heat that not only do cows run a core temperature of 38.5°C, but our Welsh Blacks where I live can happily chew the cud on a Welsh hill in horizontal snow. They have a personal central heating system.

Better still, fibre is fermented to short chain fatty acids (energetically this costs us nothing) and these are easily converted to ketones – the most efficient fuel to power our mitochondria. Tuck into that linseed bread and linseed porridge (see our *PK Cookbook)* and top up with green vegetables for free heat and fuel.

I can hear the athletes objecting to the above – a gut full of fibre will weigh them down. However, Nature comes to the rescue – at the prospect of action, adrenalin is poured out and the gut empties; this brown trouser effect[†] gives us the best of both worlds.

So, there you are – you really can get something for nothing. Apparently, amongst the eight Yorkshire phrases least understood by

Americans is:

> *And if ever thou does owt fer nowt – allus do it fer thissen'*
> *(And if you ever do anything for nothing—always do it for yourself.)*

So, maybe we can now say:

> *Thou canst get summat fer nowt – allus do it*
> *fer thissen – EZ watter, by gum!*

[†]For our American friends who may not understand the brown trousers reference the phrase derives from a desire to hide a situation where one has crapped one' trousers/pants.

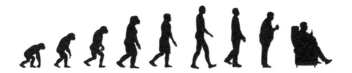

PART
3

ENERGY EXPENDITURE

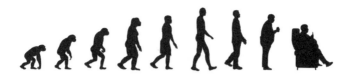

CHAPTER
12

THE BARE NECESSITIES

HOUSEKEEPING OR BASAL METABOLISM

Look for the bare necessities
The simple bare necessities
Forget about your worries and your strife
I mean the bare necessities
Old Mother Nature's recipes
That bring the bare necessities of life

Baloo the Bear* in *The Jungle Book* by Joseph Rudyard Kipling,
1865 – 1936

*Literary note: There is much variation as to which type of bear Baloo is depicted as. It seems that Kipling 'meant' Baloo to be a sloth bear and, while in the 1967 Walt Disney film version, Baloo was indeed portrayed this way, in the Russian version, he is portrayed as an Asian black bear and in live-action television shows in the US, Baloo was often portrayed by an American black bear. It seems that the Cold War even affected the identity of Baloo.

Simply staying alive requires energy – and a lot of it. Roughly two thirds of all the energy generated in the body goes on keeping the home fires burning. What this means is that we have one third of all energy generated to spend mentally and physically and much of this has to go on work to earn a living. That may not leave much for having fun – exercise, socialising and hobbies. Indeed, as we age and the energy bucket shrinks, often these are the first expenditures that are discarded – we lapse into a state of work and rest, which is no fun at all. We watch children play and marvel at their energy – but not only do they have more efficient energy delivery mechanisms, but they do not have to spend energy on work; they can spend it all on play (assuming the perfect childhood environment of benign neglect).

Let us look at where energy for basal metabolism is being spent and see how we can make this more efficient.

Where are we spending energy and why?

The energy-hungry liver

The liver spends 27% of all the energy we generate – that is, almost half of our housekeeping allowance. This is just a little more than the brain and heart combined. In terms of complexity, I think the liver ranks third below the brain and immune system. It has many unenviable jobs (at least 500 and counting) and they all require energy to fulfil, including:

- Sorting out the toxic soup that comes from the gut via the portal vein – We have a circulation within a circulation: the venous blood from the gut does not return directly to the heart, but first goes to the liver. This is just as well. Without the liver interposed to clean up the blood we would fall unconscious; indeed, this is exactly what happens in people with liver failure. So, what are the nasties that the liver has to deal with? In order of priority I suspect these are:

a) **Sugar and carbs**: Carbohydrate-based diets mean that there will be times when large amounts of glucose, fructose, sucrose and other sugars flood into the portal vein. Sugar is extremely damaging and cannot be allowed to spill over into the main circulation. The liver acts as a sponge to mop up sugar. It transforms it into glycogen and fat for storage, and this requires energy. If blood sugar levels fall, then the reverse happens and glycogen is released from storage as glucose. This too requires energy. By contrast, fat is non-toxic. So much so that it does not even need to be processed in the liver. Fats from the gut pass directly into the lymphatics and from there into the systemic circulation for immediate use as a fuel. A high-fat diet reduces the work of the liver.

b) **Toxins from the fermenting gut**: As you have read in Chapter 6, the fermenting upper gut is a toxic gut, producing alcohols, acetones, D lactates, ammonias, hydrogen sulphides and more – cripes, even the names are enough to poison me – which all spill over into the portal vein where the tolerant liver has to deal with them. This is why I think of the liver as Mother.

c) **Bacteria, fungi and viruses (so called bacteriophages) from the gut**: At medical school during the 1970s I was taught that the gut is full of microbes and there they stay. Wrong! We now know that microbes easily spill over into the bloodstream and this is called 'bacterial translocation'. We have two types of microbe that can potentially present problems. The bulk of these will be 'friendly' bacteria fermenting fibre in our lower gut. These have been an issue for millions of years, in which time we have learned to live with them and the liver is well able to deal with them – they do not cause disease and are excreted in urine. So much so that a urine infection is defined as 'more than 10,000 bacteria per ml of urine'. A one-litre pee may contain up to 10 million microbes. Problems arise with evolutionarily recent microbes from the abnormal upper fermenting gut. These have flourished with recent high-carb diets. Immune Kuppfer cells in the liver identify these and kill them before they can spread, but this demands energy.

Clinical pearl[†]: simply brushing your teeth will cause bacteraemia (bacteria in the blood) and this is why dentists insist on patients with bad hearts pre-treating with antibiotics before any dental procedure to prevent infections of the heart.

---

d) **Endotoxins and mycotoxins**: Bacteria and fungi produce their own toxins called endotoxins and mycotoxins respectively. These may be very nasty compounds, such as botulinum toxin which paralyses, and ochratoxin which causes renal failure.

e) **Infections:** Most infections get into the body via the gut. Even those microbes we inhale get stuck on to sticky mucus in our airways, drop into our oesophagus or are coughed up and swallowed into our stomach. Many are killed by stomach acid or the immune system in our gut wall, but the next line of defence is the liver where again the immune Kuppfer cells swing into action. If the liver is Mother, then the immune system must be Father – at its best when dormant but jolly useful when there is a battle to be fought! However, often he

[†]Medical aside: There is an interesting study from 2009 of 'clinical pearls' (that is 'pearls of wisdom') by Martin Lorin et al, in which Lorin states that: 'Clinical pearls are best defined as small bits of free-standing, clinically relevant information based on experience or observation.' In Maths, we call them 'tricks' and they 'shortcut' us to elegant solutions. Craig.

gets things wrong with allergy and autoimmunity (sorry Craig)

f) **Pollutants**: It is the job of the liver to deal with the toxins of the modern polluted world. These include:

- social addictions (carbs, caffeine, nicotine, alcohol and others)

- prescription drugs

- environmental pollutants

- food additives (colourings, flavourings, preservatives, pesticide residues).

All the above substances require raw materials (vitamins, minerals and amino acids) and energy to render them safe. Indeed, the liver will ramp up the levels of enzymes necessary to detox efficiently. These can be measured as part of standard liver function blood tests. Many of us are aware that drinking too much alcohol will increase levels of GGT (gamma glutamyl transferase) because this is the enzyme needed to detoxify alcohol. Other liver enzymes, such as AST (aspartate transaminase) and ALT (alanine amino transferase), may also be induced by toxic loads. Flip this on its head and we can see that high levels of these enzymes mean the liver is dealing with a toxic load. In looking for a healthy liver I do not simply want to see levels of enzymes outside of reference ranges, I want to see them as low as possible.

Clinical pearl: Levels of GGT, AST, ALT and bilirubin predict longevity – the lower the better. High levels reflect high toxic loads.

---

g) **Recycling lactic acid when we over-do things**: Lactic acid is a major problem for my CFS and ME patients and an increasing problem for my ageing patients. Many are constantly pushing the energy boundaries. The result is that to do what they want or need to do, they switch into anaerobic (without oxygen) metabolism which produces lactic acid. CFS and ME sufferers and athletes know all about this substance – it is very painful. The production of lactic acid provides the body with two molecules of energy-supplying ATP (see page 82). However, to clear this painful particle back to pyruvate requires six molecules of ATP from the liver. Whilst a switch into anaerobic metabolism may be a lifesaving tool to escape predation, one then has a greedy energy payback.[‡] This really is a case of short-term gain, long-term pain.

Clinical pearl: High levels of lactate dehydrogenase (LDH) in the blood predict a shorter life. Athletes who over-train will also have high levels of LDH; they may be fit but they are not healthy.

---

h) **Plant toxins**: If you look at life from the point of view of a plant, it does not want to be eaten. It cannot, like an animal, run away. What it can do is to render itself as poisonous as possible so it either

---

[‡] A friend of mine is an Olympic rower. He describes the climax of a race. Most of the race is conducted in aerobic metabolism when oxygen use parallels oxygen delivery. Towards the end there is a sprint finish, and this is achieved through anaerobic means. There is massive production of lactic acid which is extremely painful – much mental over-ride is needed to ignore this pain to carry on. The most energy-demanding part of the body is the retina and the brain. As oxygen falls in the blood, vision starts to go, and the brain starts to shut down. Peripheral vision is lost at first and things close down until all Sam can see is a receding dot of light. The aim is to lose consciousness as you cross the finishing line – anything less and you have not timed your sprint well enough!

tastes dreadful or renders the consumer acutely ill. Many of these poisons are lectins and these are not just toxic to humans but also to microbes. Indeed, lectins are plant antibiotics. The snowdrop lectin is particularly toxic and, of course, poisonous to humans. It has been investigated for use in chemical warfare.[§]

Clinical pearl: The liver is highly adaptive – it will detoxify using the 'cheapest' route. About 10% of the population have Gilbert's syndrome which means one route of detoxification ('glucuronidation' for the biochemists) does not work. The liver can employ other routes, but these are more energy-expensive and demanding of raw materials. It will, therefore, be no surprise to learn that these slow detoxifiers often suffer fatigue because they are more susceptible to poisonings.[¶] Bilirubin is detoxified slowly, and Gilbert's is defined by a bilirubin of more than 19 mg/dl. Jaundice appears at levels above 30 mg/dl. I like to see levels below 10 mg/dl. If you have a bilirubin above 10 then you should take glutathione 250 mg for life.

[§]**Footnote**: The potato is particularly sensitive to blight and insect attack, which means crops are heavily sprayed with pesticide. Some bright spark decided to use genetic modification to cross a snowdrop with a potato to render it resistant to blight. By 1998 this GMO potato was within a few weeks of marketing. Rowett Institute scientist Arpad Pusztai was asked to see if these potatoes were safe for human consumption. He found these snowdrop-potatoes were, like snowdrops, highly toxic. To prevent an industry cover-up, he appeared in a *World in Action* interview and stated: 'The rats in my experiments suffered stunted growth and had suppressed immune systems...'. He further stated of the snowdrop-potato cross, 'If you gave me the choice now, I wouldn't eat it'. He considered that by feeding such... 'Well it would be very, very unfair to use our fellow citizens as guinea pigs'. Because of his work, this snowdrop-potato cross was not marketed but Pusztai was sacked from his job. In 2005 he received a whistle-blower award from the Federation of German Scientists. Now that is what I call a good man.

i) **Making bile** to allow fats to be emulsified prior to absorption from the gut, and to excrete toxins such as bilirubin (this is what stains our turds brown).

j) Making proteins for blood clotting and for immune function.

> **Clinical pearl**: A good level of albumin is a marker for longevity. The reference range is 34-50 g/l with 50 being good.

k) And many other jobs.

***Footnote**: In 1999 I was involved in a group action of farmers poisoned by organophosphate pesticides. Exposures were from sheep dip, from handling grain (all is treated with organophosphate whilst in storage), from organophosphates used in the milking parlour for fly control and organophosphates used as crop sprays. One sufferer was a government inspector poisoned by the fumes from previously dipped sheep up for sale in sheep markets. It was notable that 14 of the 27 farmers also had Gilbert's syndrome. Subsequent work by Professor Nicola Cherry showed that about a third of the farming population were slow detoxifiers and this predisposed them to the pathological sequaelae of chronic organophosphate poisoning – chronic fatigue syndromes, premature ageing and chronic disease. Furthermore, Professor Rosemary Waring demonstrated that people with Parkinson's disease were also slow detoxifiers.

$^{\#}$**Classical mythological note**: Tantalus was a rich but wicked king of Sipylus. He once tried to serve his own son as a delicacy at a feast with the Gods. This was beyond the pale even for Zeus, who punished him to go forever thirsty and hungry in Hades despite being placed in a pool of water and almost within reach of a fruit tree. For Tantalus, the symptom of thirst was to remind him of his wickedness and suffer for it rather than a genuine need to drink water.

The energy-hungry kidneys

The kidneys are so demanding of an absolutely constant supply of energy that the body has evolved a hormonal system (the renin-angiotensin system) to make sure they continue to be perfused with blood when all around is failing. Kidneys first filter blood in the glomeruli (microscopic tubules that perform for this purpose), then scavenge the precious salts, amino acids and sugars that leak through. This process demands much energy.

Clinical pearl: Some of the worst nourished I see are those that think it is a good idea to drink lots of water. Problems arise because whilst we can drink pure water, we cannot pee pure water – inevitably some mineral salts are washed out. This situation is made much worse by diuretics and doctors. Diuretics work by inhibiting salt scavenging – the osmotic effect of salt pulls water and so large volumes of pee (salts and water) are lost. This problem is compounded by the doctors who advise their patients to avoid salt when the correct advice is to take more salt and all other minerals in proportion. Indeed, this is why I developed my Sunshine salt – the perfect rehydrating mix.

Athletes have been endlessly advised to drink water prophylactically 'before they become thirsty', but this is nonsense. We get the symptoms of thirst for very good reasons.[#] If we follow this advice, we end up with under-performing, waterlogged athletes.

The energy-hungry brain

It may account for only 2% of body weight but the brain is vastly demanding of energy and uses 20% of all that is generated. We can reduce energy delivery by many means – restrict the fuel supply, restrict the oxygen supply, develop hypothyroidism to name a few – but the end results are the same – a foggy brain, acute confusional states, dementia, loss of consciousness and death.

We know from our own experience that the brain needs much energy. Those in jobs demanding of mental and emotional work will be exhausted by the end of the day. I love seeing patients but am shattered by 5 pm; by contrast, I can work in my garden for eight hours without tiring. We can make lifestyle changes to reduce the mental work of the brain but what is much more difficult to deal with is the emotional hole in the energy bucket (see Chapter 13).

The heart and circulation

At rest, the heart and circulatory system spend just 7% of all energy generated by the body. The heart and muscular arteries are responsible only for getting blood to the little arteries (arterioles) just prior to the capillaries, the narrowest blood vessels. Capillary circulation is dependent on background heat (see Chapter 11). Blood is returned to the heart by the veins and one-way flow relies on valves within the veins assisted by the muscular contractions of movement and breathing.

How to reduce housekeeping energy expenditure

To make sure we have enough energy for all these demanding body systems we need to make our energy expenditure on housekeeping as efficient as possible. An understanding of the above mechanisms tells us how to minimise the bare necessities. In order of priority my view is:

1. **Eat the right diet**: The liver consumes most energy dealing with food. In order of priority eat:

   - Fat – this does not even need processing by the liver; it passes directly into the systemic bloodstream via the lymphatics

   - Fibre – this is fermented in the large bowel by friendly bacteria to produce short chain fats, a source of free fuel and heat (see Chapter 6)

   - Protein – this too needs little processing and is low in toxins.

   Indeed, my very sickest patients do best on a 'GAPs' diet based on meat, fat, bone broths, eggs and fish. The most nutritious (and so delicious) food of course is liver.**

   - Organic raw (or lightly boiled/steamed) above-ground (i.e. low-carbohydrate) vegetables
   - No starchy carbs as there is potential for them to ferment (see Chapter 6).
   - None of the major allergens – that is, dairy products and gluten.

2. **Give the liver the raw materials to do its job most efficiently**: These include all the B vitamins, vitamin C, many minerals, essential fatty acids and glutathione (250 mg daily). See Appendix I for doses.

3. **Reduce the chemical burden**: Avoid social drugs, prescription drugs, food additives and eat as organically as is possible.

**Organ meats were highly prized by primitive man – the chief hunter would receive the heart, brain, glands and bone marrow, lesser hunters ate organ meats and the rubbish was given to the women who, poor things, had to eat rib eye, sirloin and rump steak.

4. **Do not overeat**: This is much easier once you are off your addictive foods. The average USA consumer purchases 250% of the calories they need (shamefully much is thrown away).

5. **Take vitamin C** to bowel tolerance (explained on page 177). This multitasks to prevent the upper fermenting gut (see page 108), prevent infection, detoxify and mop up free radicals (see Appendix 5).

6. **Keep warm**: Sunbathe whenever possible (see Chapter 11).

7. **Detoxify**: Once a week use a heating regime to reduce the load of chemicals you are carrying in storage (see Chapter 13 and the next section).

Heating regimes to detox

We live in a polluted world. It is impossible to avoid all pollutants. I often do analyses on fat samples and I have yet to see a 'normal' (toxin free) result. The best that can be done is to keep your body burden as low as possible and hope that your liver will deal with the rest.

Broadly speaking we have three categories of toxin to deal with:

1. Toxins that are water soluble will get into the bloodstream and pass through the liver and kidneys to be excreted.

2. Toxins that get stuck in organs such as the heart, brain and bone marrow. Largely speaking these are heavy metals.[††]

[††]Footnote: During the Gulf War depleted uranium (DU) was used in warheads to give them tank-busting capability. DU vapourised in the explosions and so could be inhaled by frontline troops. It tends to be deposited in bones and there it sticks. In response to the concerns of Gulf War veterans, the MoD arranged for some to have urine tests. These were normal – of course! DU is stuck in bone – not excreted – and there it remains for life.

3. Persistent organic pollutants (POPs) that bio-accumulate in fat. The most commonly encountered POPs are organochlorine pesticides, such as DDT, industrial chemicals, most notably polychlorinated biphenyls (PCB), as well as unintentional by-products of many industrial processes, especially polychlorinated dibenzo-p-dioxins (PCDD) and dibenzofurans (PCDF), commonly known as 'dioxins'. They are ubiquitously present and unavoidable. When I do tests on fat samples the results come back in milligrams per kilogram. By contrast, blood levels are reported in micrograms per kilogram – there is a thousand-fold difference. Human fat is toxic.

Clinical pearl: Weight loss can cause acute poisoning since POPs are mobilised from fat into the blood stream. Arguably any weight loss regime should be accompanied by heating regimes to mitigate the poisoning. The converse may be true – as we are poisoned the body may lay down fat deliberately to mitigate the effects of such toxicity. This ploy is used in intensively reared farm animals where those fed on inorganic foods and antibiotic gain weight faster than their organic contemporaries.

One of the nastiest organochlorines is the carcinogen lindane. It has been banned... except for the sugar beet industry for sugar production. This is big in Lincolnshire and so is breast cancer.

Heating regimes for detoxing

Early on in my career I was aware of a study by Dr William Rea demonstrating the effectiveness of heating regimes to get rid of POPs. However, I wanted to know just how effective they were. I started to collect data before and after heating regimes and learned much.

The critical facts were:

- It does not matter which heating regime is used – they are all effective. If you are fit enough to exercise, then do so. If you are unwell and cannot, then the far-infrared saunas are tolerated best. If, like me, you are lazy but well, then traditional saunas and steam baths are great. Spa therapy such as a hot bath, enhanced by Epsom salts (500 g in 68 litres of water) also works well. I love them all! The effect of all the aforementioned are enhanced by massage.

- The idea is the heat mobilises POPs from the subcutaneous fat on the superficial fatty layer of the skin whence they can be washed off. It is not necessary to sweat for these heating regimes to be effective, but the washing off after is as important as the heating.

- Levels of POPs come down exponentially. So, 50 heatings will halve the load (to 50%), a further 50 halve it again (to 25%). A further 50 to 12.5% and so on… You will never get rid of every molecule.

- Some who are very toxic will be made worse initially as some of the POPs will be mobilised throughout the body. Start with low heats and short times to mitigate this effect.

One family I tested had all been poisoned by organophosphates used in a house fumigation. Men doing the work all wore chemical warfare suits and breathing apparatus, but the family were told it was safe to return in 24 hours. They all became acutely ill and fat samples showed they had all been poisoned by the same organophosphate. Thankfully it was an RB family.[‡‡] They travelled to Danubius spa in Budapest and underwent daily regimes of spa, sauna and massage for three weeks. They returned and requested repeat testing. 'No, no...' I said, '...far too soon'. But I was wrong – tests showed the organophosphates were now undetectable.

I have come to the view that we should all be doing some sort of heating regime on a weekly basis.

And let us not forget that such heating regimes have stood the test of time. The Romans bathed a lot. It was almost a daily thing, and this applied across a wide variety of social classes. For the RB Romans ('patricians'), bathing was a refined and deeply social event and involved a ritual of successive forms of bathing. First, one entered the apodyterium where one undressed and left one's clothes. Then it was into the tepidarium (warm room), and from there into the caldarium (hot room) for a steam. Finally, the RB Roman would enter the frigidarium (cold room) with its tank of cold water. Then the bather would return to tepidarium for a massage with oils and a final scraping with metal implements. Some baths also contained a laconium (dry, resting room) where the bather completed the process by resting and sweating. Mixed bathing was at times commonplace and at other times frowned upon depending on the fad at the time, but the bathhouse usually had three entrances: one for men, one for women, and one for slaves, who were brought along to service the RBs.

[‡‡] **Footnote**: I have used the term 'RB' after reading an article about a merchant bank who decided to target their hundred wealthiest clients for a new investment scheme. A minion was detailed to organise the letters using mail merge. Unfortunately for him, he forgot to replace the mail merge name with the clients' real name. This meant they all received a letter which opened: ; '*Dear Rich Bastard*'.

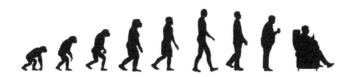

CHAPTER
13

ENERGY EXPENDITURE

THE IMMUNOLOGICAL HOLE IN
THE ENERGY BUCKET

There's a hole in the bucket, dear Liza, dear Liza,
There's a hole in the bucket, dear Liza, a hole.

Then fix it, dear Henry, dear Henry, dear Henry,
Then fix it, dear Henry, dear Henry, fix it.

With what shall I fix it, dear Liza, dear Liza?
With what shall I fix it, dear Liza, with what?

Read this book dear Henry, dear Henry, dear Henry,
*Read this book, dear Henry, dear Henry, read it!**

Historical note: The earliest known version of this song seems to be from the German collection of songs *Bergliederbüchlein* (c 1700) and recounts a dialogue between a woman named Liese, and an unnamed man.

The immune system

The immune system is our standing army which, at rest, should consume little energy. Of course, we want it to leap into action to deal with acute infection. In this event we may run a fever and develop symptoms such as mucus production, coughing and sneezing to expel and kill the invaders. This process we call inflammation and needs much energy – so much so that a fit and healthy young person, given a dose of flu, may become bedbound. As is well recognised, this is always much more severe for men.[†]

For those interested in the phenomenon of 'man flu', an article in the *British Medical Journal* discusses, and I quote, 'whether men are wimps or just have weaker immune systems.'[1] The problem for us all – men and women – is that Western lifestyles and diet put us into a pro-inflammatory state which is both damaging and energy consuming. Let's look at the mechanisms.

The fermenting upper gut

Altogether 90% of the immune system is associated with the gut to keep the microbes in the fermenting gut at bay. However, high-carbohydrate diets lead to fermentation in the upper gut (stomach and small intestine) with a build-up of unfriendly bacteria and yeasts. These too must be kept at bay and that needs more energy.

Professor Rosemary Waring, Reader in Human Toxicology at the University of Birmingham, UK, asked the fascinating question, where in their bodies do wild animals store fat when food is plentiful? She collected the specimens from road-kill whilst cycling to work. Animals

---

[†] To quote an internet meme: '*Full recovery from Man-Flu will take place much quicker if their simple requests for care, sympathy and regular cups of tea are met. Is that really so much to ask? Florence Nightingale would have done it.*'

dump fat where immune cells are concentrated – namely, around lymph nodes. This makes perfect sense – infection is a common killer and the immune cells need a local and ready supply of fuel to fight it. This explains the beer belly of high-carb consumers – they have an upper fermenting gut and fat is deposited there to fuel the immune system to prevent invasion of the bloodstream and septicaemia. (Guess what? We are currently seeing epidemics of septicaemia (or sepsis)!)

Microbial translocation

The gut is full of microbes and there they stay. Wrong. Some spill over into the bloodstream and this is called 'bacterial translocation'. Most will pass through the kidneys and be excreted, but some get stuck in other tissue, such as muscles and joints. The immune cells attack and inflammation with degeneration results. We know that metabolic syndrome is the major risk factor for arthritis and osteoporosis.

Allergy and autoimmunity

Allergy and autoimmunity are useless and destructive forms of inflammation that occur when the immune system is inappropriately switched on. This occurs by mistake and one example of how this can happen is through vaccination. The idea of vaccination is to temporarily switch on inflammation against the microbe contained within such so that the immune cells learn to recognise the enemy in the future. Good idea – but the immune system is not dull; it will not recognise and not be activated by the dead or inactive microbes used in vaccines. For vaccination to work, a wake-up call is needed from an 'adjuvant'. Such adjuvants include mercury, aluminium, neomycin, squalene and other similar nasties. These are very good at switching on inflammation; unfortunately for some, this does not then switch off again. Clinically we experience this as allergy and/or autoimmunity. Both are common, affecting possibly 40% and 20% of Westerners respectively.

In my own experience, I see many patients with myalgic encephalitis (ME – chronic fatigue syndrome AND inflammation) following vaccination, especially after HPV vaccination. We also know pollution can switch on allergy and a good example of this came from a study which showed that hay fever was more common in the city despite pollen counts being lowest there.[2] The reason? Diesel particulates were sticking to grass pollen and acting as an adjuvant to switch on the immune system in the airways. There are many other pollutants that have this adjuvant (provoking) action.

Chronic infection

You and I represent a free lunch for any microbe that is able to make itself at home in our warm, moist, delicious bodies where they can be very comfortable and enjoy free sex for the procreation of their selfish genes. As we age, we risk acquiring new infections and these drive pathologies. This is the subject of our book *The Infection Game – Life is an Arms Race*.

Every major pathology for Westerners, from diabetes and dementia to cancer and coronaries, has an infectious associate. All these conditions are associated with inflammation and fatigue. The converse is also true – those people with poor energy delivery mechanisms and inflammations have a greatly increased risk of these nasty killers. Chronic infection often starts with an acute infection that is poorly dealt with. Improving our immune defences is therefore a vital part of survival.

Strategies to counteract inflammation

With a clear understanding of mechanisms, we can put in place strategies to prevent the pro-inflammatory states I've described. These strategies are just the starting points; there is much more detail in our books *The Infection Game* and *Ecological Medicine – the antidote to Big Pharma and Fast Food*.

1. Put the body into such a healthy state that microbes cannot move in.

2. Prepare now, and stock the tools you will need, to deal with the unexpected, inevitable and overwhelming microbial attacks. With these tools, mass vaccination becomes irrelevant.

3. Act now to avoid and get rid of those pollutants that switch on allergy and autoimmunity.

4. Identify and address chronic infections which you may currently be carrying; the older and the sicker you are the more likely this is to be the case.

1. Put the body into such a healthy state that microbes cannot move in

Diabetes is often picked up as a diagnosis when there are recurrent infections. The mechanism here is that sugar oozes onto the skin resulting in spots and boils, into urine resulting in UTIs and into the airways resulting in coughs and colds. The single most important strategy is not to give microbes a free lunch. Yes, sigh, all roads lead to Rome,‡ or in the case of health, the PK diet with a few supplementary vitamins and minerals (see Appendix 1); this is non-negotiable. (See also the Groundhog regimes in Appendices 2, 3 and 4.)

To quote Linus Pauling (1901-1994), the only person to win two unshared Nobel prizes in two different scientific fields: 'People who take these vitamins … .in the optimum amounts can live 25 or 35 years longer than otherwise. More than that, they will be free of diseases. This optimum nutrition… cuts down the probability of developing cancer, or heart disease or diabetes, or infectious diseases.'

Prepare now, and stock up with the two tools, iodine and vitamin C, you will need to deal with the unexpected, inevitable and overwhelming microbial attacks. With these tools, mass vaccination becomes irrelevant.

Iodine

To quote Dr David Derry: 'Though iodine kills all pathogens on the skin within 90 seconds, its use as an antibiotic/antiviral/antifungal has been completely ignored by modern medicine. Iodine is by far the best antibiotic, antiviral and antiseptic of all time.'[3] Why so? I ask. Follow the money!

- Iodine contact-kills all microbes. Purchase Lugol's iodine 15%. Drizzle this on to any cuts, grazes, superficial burns or insect bites to prevent infection. Lugol's gets rid of fungal infections, cold sores, shingles, chicken pox, verrucas, spots, boils or nail infections. Apply neat Lugol's once – it stings a bit, but no pain, no gain. Then move to iodine oil (see next) to top up. I always carry Lugol's iodine in my pocket for such emergencies.

- Iodine oil is a mixture of coconut oil, 10 parts, to Lugol's 15%, one part. It is great for more general and widespread application

‡**Classical note**: 'All roads lead to Rome'is a proverb in many languages and most likely derives from the *Milliarium Aureum* (the 'Golden Milestone'). The Golden Milestone was a monument (made from marble or gilded bronze) erected by Emperor Caesar Augustus in the central Forum of Ancient Rome. All roads were considered to begin at this monument and all distances in the Roman Empire were measured relative to it.

for eczema (which is very often driven by infection), rosacea, psoriasis, perineal infections, cradle cap, dermatitis and, indeed, almost any skin pathology.

- Inhaled iodine contact-kills all cold and influenza viruses. Put 2 drops of Lugol's 15% into a salt pipe and sniff 15-20 times until the iodine smell has gone. Iodine is volatile and this method treats all upper and lower respiratory infections, acute and chronic. I now have two patients with bronchiectasis who have been antibiotic-free for over a year.

Vitamin C

Vitamin C also contact-kills all microbes. The key is the dose. For this reason, it has consistently failed the 'does it prevent colds' test. The dose is individual and varies from person to person, with age, diet, season and infectious load. Ascorbic acid is the cheapest and best form of vitamin C and it needs to be taken to bowel tolerance (BT). The idea here is that the body will use whatever vitamin C it requires – and those requirements extend from perfect antioxidant status, reducing toxic load, preventing upper fermenting gut to dealing with any systemic load of infection. Indeed, one's bowel tolerance dose is a good clinical gauge of one's state of health. My favourite quote is from Dr Frederick Robert Klenner, BS MS FCCP, FAAFP (1907 – 1984): '*The patient should get large doses of vitamin C in all pathological conditions while the physician ponders the diagnosis.*'

My view is that we should all be taking BT doses of vitamin C all the time. We need to dose little and often through the day. I reckon those in perfect health, on a PK diet with no fermenting gut, need 5-10 grams for optimal health. Put this dose in your daily bottle of water and slurp through the day. If you slightly over-dose, and this is necessary initially to determine your bowel tolerance, you may get foul-smelling wind, then loose bowel motions. This occurs if not all the vitamin C is absorbed and that remaining in the guts starts to kill off some of the friendly bacteria in the lower gut which are then fermented by other friendlies... definitely an experiment for the weekend!

There is more detail in Appendix 5. BT is the dose you arrive at by increasing your dose of vitamin C daily to a level at which you have diarrhoea and then reducing the dose down to just below that diarrhoea-inducing dose.

2. Act now to avoid and get rid of those pollutants that switch on allergy and autoimmunity

You must AVOID, in order of priority, all the following. This advice is based on clinical problems I have seen triggered by these issues:

- Vaccination – As I mentioned above, HPV vaccine appears to be particularly effective in triggering serious disease as detailed in Christina England's book *Shattered Dreams*. In the follow up trials of this vaccine, death is underwhelmingly described as a 'serious adverse effect'.

- Dental amalgam – In November 2003 I chaired a scientific meeting of the British Society for Environmental Medicine at the Royal College of General Practitioners. At this I was woken up to the dangers of mercury following a lecture by Professor Fritz Lorscheide. He showed how mercury evaporates from dental amalgam, is inhaled and is deposited in the brain. There it disrupts tubulin, the self-assembling loo-roll-shaped protein that protects nerve fibres. As a result, nerve fibres contract into a neurofibrillary tangle. This is the pathological hallmark of Alzheimer's disease. I trotted off to get all my dental amalgam removed.

- Mycotoxins from water damaged buildings – A scientific paper by Dr Joseph Brewer has shown that over 90% of CFS/ME sufferers test positive for mycotoxins.[4] Professor Tamara Tuuminen has shown that mould and mycotoxin exposure result in symptoms which 'include recurrent infections, chronic rhinosinusitis, swelling of the sinuses, irritation of the eyes and skin, voice problems, chronic non-productive cough, neurological symptoms, joint and muscle symptoms, irritable bowel syndrome and cognitive problems. Underdiagnosed or neglected continuous insidious inflammation may lead to Myalgic Encephalitis/Chronic Fatigue Syndrome (ME/CFS) especially when trigged by new infections or even vaccination.[5]

- Prescription and social drugs – These mask symptoms and are often addictive.

- Air pollution – especially smoking, industrial discharges, diesel fumes and pesticide spray drift. The late Dr Dick van Steenis showed how people living close to polluting industry, such as power stations, chemicals and cement works, oil refineries and waste disposal sites, increased their risk of cancer, cardiovascular disease and birth defects – the nearer the polluting source the greater the risk.

- Conventionally (non-organic) grown and GM foods – The most used pesticide is glyphosate, and most GMO crops are modified for glyphosate resistance – that is, you can use even more of the stuff in growing those crops. Glyphosate is present in almost all foodstuffs that are not organically grown.[§]

- Electromagnetic pollution – All the evidence is showing that 5-G is a serious health hazard. Professor Martin Pall tells us that the roll out of 5-G constitutes a massive, uncontrolled 'health experiment' for these reasons:

- Networks will transmit data 100 times faster using shorter radiation waves

- It is biologically plausible that cell-phone radiation is carcinogenic

- The health effects of new shorter millimeter waves used in 5-G have hardly been studied.

- **Silicones used in surgery** – These may be perceived by the body as a foreigner and so be subject to immune attack. The problem is that silicone is a plastic and is such a tough molecule that no biological enzymes can break it down. Immune cells can launch a full attack to try to 'kill' the silicone but this is ineffective. Silicone thus may switch on localised, or perhaps a more general, inflammation. I reckon I have seen over 250 sick women following breast implants. This often starts with hardening and tenderness of the breast followed by more systemic inflammation that results in the clinical pictures of fibromyalgia, chronic fatigue and autoimmunity. I have one patient whose hard silicone implant was treated by 'external capsulotomy' – the surgeon crushed the breast between his hands until the implant ruptured. Yes, this 'softened' the lump, but silicone spread into the armpit, down the chest wall and a massive immune reaction resulted. Kath now has what feels like

§ **Footnote**: Monsanto/Bayer have just lost another court case showing their product, Roundup, (glyphosate) caused Dewayne Johnson's cancer. The two issues at stake were, first, did Monsanto's product cause Johnson's terminal cancer and, second, did Monsanto fail to warn consumers that its product is potentially harmful. In both cases, the jury's answer was a resounding 'yes'. This led to Monsanto's being ordered to pay $39 million in 'compensatory damages', covering the medical expenses, suffering, lost wages and other expenses caused by his illness. On top of that, the jury added: 'punitive damages' of $250 million—which Monsanto was ordered to pay as punishment for knowingly selling a product that is harmful.

bunches of grapes under her skin and, of course, chronic pain. The surgeons dare not operate because these lumps surround the brachial plexus – such surgery would risk a paralysed arm.

- **Metals used in surgery** – These too are foreign bodies and can likewise activate the immune system and again cannot be 'digested' away. They may switch on localised, followed by more systemic, inflammation. Nickel is the worst offender but increasingly we are seeing allergies to chromium, cobalt and titanium. It has been estimated that about 1% of joint replacements may result in further disease. One of my patients was a very intelligent and on-the-ball 85-year-old who underwent minor surgery to correct a hammer toe. Metal was used. The surgery was a technical success. However, six weeks later she developed local pain and inflammation, not due to infection, that spread up her leg. A few months later she developed generalised arthritis. During this time her personality changed, and she became increasingly anxious, and lacking in her usual self-confidence. I arranged lymphocyte sensitivity tests[*] which showed a high reaction to the very metals used in her surgery – namely chromium, nickel and titanium. She has now deteriorated, over 18 months, into a full-blown dementia. The surgeons refuse to remove the metal from her foot.

- **Cosmetics** – especially perfumes and hair dyes. Hair dyes are known carcinogens. They are one of the commonest findings when I do tests of toxicity. The only safe hair dye is henna, but just because it says 'henna' on the bottle does not mean it is safe! Only natural henna is okay.

[*]**Note**, such metal sensitivity tests are available from www.melisa.org/

- **Household cleaners** – If you can smell something then it is in your brain – the olfactory nerve is an extension of the brain.

- **Plasticisers** – The problem with these chemicals was flagged up by neonatologists working with premature babies in intensive care who were dying without obvious reason. These babies often have endotracheal tubes, umbilical catheters, nasogastric tubes and nasal cannulae fitted. Phthalate metabolites were detected even in the first urine samples of very low birth-weight newborns. Phthalate levels were higher in the first weeks of intensive invasive procedures and in preterm infants with a birth weight less than 1000 grams. Phthalates are known endocrine disrupters. As a result of this research, all plastics used in ITU must now be phthalate free.

You must also GET RID of nasties that have accumulated over time:

- **VOCs and other such toxins** – Heating regimes are effective in getting rid of all pollutants except metals. Because we live in such a toxic world and many are unavoidable, we should all be doing a weekly heating regime followed by a shower to wash off the nasties. Those with the energy can exercise hard, otherwise saunaing, hot bath or sunbathing are ideal. (See Chapter 12 for more details.)

- **Toxic metals** – These get stuck in tissues and must be dislodged. Much good can be achieved with taking friendly minerals which displace the toxic minerals, then taking glutathione (250 mg daily) to grab the toxins for excretion. (Again, see Chapter 12.)

- **Chronic infections** – Identify and address any chronic infections which you may currently be carrying. As I have said, the older and the sicker you are, the more likely it is that you have some on board. As we age, we should all put in place Groundhog Chronic (Appendix 4). Indeed, this is the starting point to treat all chronic infection and all chronic disease. If, having established this regimen, you are still not well, you need further medical investigation. There is much more detail in *The Infection Game* and *Ecological Medicine*. Practitioners who can guide you through this process can be found at https://naturalhealthworldwide.com/

Conclusion

In summary then, we fix the immunological hole in the energy bucket by:

- avoiding things that cause an immune response
- getting rid of things (toxins) we already have that are causing it, and
- addressing any chronic infections that may be making the hole bigger.

Unlike Henry, we will not go around in circles, unable to fix this hole in a classic deadlock situation, whereby in order to fix his bucket's hole he (thinks he) needs a bucket with no hole. We have the tools to mend it, and these are available to all. Again, just do it!

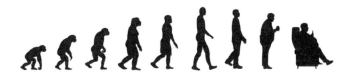

CHAPTER
14

ENERGY EXPENDITURE

THE EMOTIONAL HOLE IN THE
ENERGY BUCKET

I don't want to be at the mercy of my emotions. I want to use them,
to enjoy them, and to dominate them.

The Picture of Dorian Gray, Oscar Wilde, 1854 – 1900

Like many things that Oscar Wilde said, controlling your emotions
is easier said than done, but that is no reason not to try. The further
you get with closing the emotional hole in your energy bucket, the
better you will feel.

How energy is generated in the brain

What is fascinating about the brain is that its cells do not have the
numbers of mitochondria to explain its vast energy requirements.
There has to be another 'energy supplier' to explain this discrepancy.

121

At medical school we were taught that the myelin sheath that wraps itself around all nerve fibres was simply insulation. Wrong! Sylvia Ravera has shown these fatty sheaths have adopted identical mitochondrial biochemistry so they can create the ATP (energy) molecule right at the point of need.[1] This energy is required for an electrical wave to run along nerve cell fibres, or 'axons'.

However, in the brain the ATP molecule has an additional job. It also multitasks as a neurotransmitter. When the electrical impulse running along the nerve axon comes to a synapse (that is, a gap where one nerve cell meets another), the message is carried to the next nerve by chemical messengers called neurotransmitters. However, for the nerve end to be able to release these neurotransmitters, ATP is required. What this means is that ATP is a co-transmitter – for any neurotransmitter to be effective, ATP needs to be present.

The mechanism appears to be that the vesicles (tiny bubbles) containing neurotransmitters at the axon tip are composed of protein polymers holding neurotransmitter bound together with sticky calcium EZ honeycomb water (see page 79 to explain this 'fourth phase' of water). A shot of ATP phosphorylates to trigger the unfolding process that releases the neurotransmitter into the synaptic space to conduct a nerve impulse. Without ATP, no transmission is possible.

This gives us a biologically plausible explanation for how poor energy delivery mechanisms can be involved in depression and dementia, and other such pathologies. It has long been accepted despite little or no experimental evidence, that depression is associated with low serotonin levels. It may simply be that the serotonin is present in the nerve vesicle but cannot be released due to lack of ATP. What this means is that the treatment of all psychological and psychiatric disorders should demand proper attention to energy delivery mechanisms.

Why the brain requires so much energy

The brain requires so much energy because:

- a great deal is required for nerve impulses

- where much energy is produced there are free radicals generated that need clearing away

- the brain is plastic and constantly breaking down and reforming connections. Indeed, throughout life the brain generates one million new connections every second.

Anxiety: a common energy-sapping symptom

Anxiety is an essential evolutionary tool for survival:

- Too little vigilance and we run into danger. In the primitive world this would have been food supply, the cold, predators and local wars in the survival of the fittest. In the modern world this translates to financial trouble.

- Too much vigilance and we waste energy with anxiety. We avoid all risk-taking situations with social isolation, driven by issues from agoraphobia to avoidance of eye contact. OCD behaviours, such as checking, locking and cleanliness rituals, reflect an illogical, inappropriate, energy-sapping avoidance of perceived, but not real, dangers.

 feel very fortunate to live in the Western world where for most he greatest concern is financial security. We do not have to worry about food, cold and predators. In my small, complex, social world all members are expert in their field and valued for such. I may be a good quack, but Angie is the best golfer and gardener, Les the best stonemason and builder, Connor the best football player, Michelle the best artist, Peter the best shot and Craig the best mathematician and writer. We can all hold our heads high, enjoy and celebrate each other's successes.

The modern world, however, via social media, has changed our tribal size* so that we no longer fit into a tribal structure. Those using social media live in a very large world where they are all judged by common themes in which failure to comply and compete is social opprobrium. Insufficient 'likes' bring the anxiety of social failure. Social media, like many addictions, is a good servant but a poor master. Social media, online gaming, mobile phones (and especially smartphones), computers and internet addiction kick an emotional hole in the energy bucket.

Anxiety about the past and future

Post-traumatic stress (PTS) of childhood or life horrors is remarkably common. Most of us have skeletons in the cupboard. Similarly, we all have anxieties about the future (the 'What if?' question). Both can be much helped by psychological techniques, but PTS can be prevented and treated by quality sleep (see Chapter 9). As you have read, it is non-REM sleep that allows us to rationalise the events of the day and REM sleep that allows us to problem-solve the events of the future. I suspect PTS is greatly on the increase because sleep has deteriorated

* 'Dunbar's number' suggests a cognitive limit to the number of people with whom you can have stable social relationships; to be a stable social relationship, you must know who each person is and you must understand all the various interactions between people in the group. This number was first arrived at by the British anthropologist, Robin Dunbar, who found a correlation between primate brain size and average social group size during his studies in the 1990s. By using the average human brain size and extrapolating the results from primates, he suggested that humans can maintain about 150 stable relationships.[2]

in quality and quantity. Sleep quality is impaired by the spiking adrenalin that follows the wobbly blood sugars of carbohydrate-based diets. If one relives the memories of the day in an adrenalin-fuelled environment, then unpleasant memories will be reinforced with nightmares and flashbacks. The starting point to treat PTS is therefore a PK diet. Success has also been seen with beta-blockers taken at night which block this action of adrenalin and allow one to rationalise nasty memories in a safe environment and tuck them away safely to be ignored. The following case history is from our book *Ecological Medicine*:

Dorothy is an ME patient. She is a qualified nurse who first consulted me in 2004, then aged 43. She had become so ill that she was bedbound, too ill to sit up and requiring full-time care. With great determination and application, she put in place all the difficult things I ask my patients to do with respect to my standard work up (PK diet, supplements, detox etc). She improved somewhat but this was not really cutting it. It was only then that her appalling history of childhood abuse and bullying came to the fore. It appals me what some parents are capable of – only yesterday I spoke to a 70-year-old who described living in fear of her violent mother. When Dad was away, she spent the night sitting with her back against the bedroom door holding a knife to protect herself. She did not realise it but of course she too was suffering from PTSD. Both she and Dorothy had been hard-wired for hypervigilance for life. This wrecks sleep and is a risk factor for much pathology. They had both experienced a trauma, in the true sense of its Greek derivative – a 'wound' – and their wounds had remained unhealed for years.

Dorothy, clever girl, equipped herself with a heart-rate

monitor, to discover that throughout sleep her heart rate was highly variable, ranging from a normal of 70 bpm up to 140 bpm. Clearly this was adrenalin-fuelled. She had a vicious self-perpetuating cycle of terrifying dreams, with outpouring of stress hormones to reinforce those vile memories. This was something over which she had no conscious control.

Sleep is such a vital part of good health. The World Health Organization has classified shift-work as a probable carcinogen. Sleep deprivation is a greater risk for accidents than being drunk. It even impacts on natural killer cells and immune function. So, for Dorothy the question was how could we change her sleep in such a way as to allow her brain to discard these destructive memories?

Simply taking hypnotics was ineffective. Although she could be rendered unconscious by such, she did not get proper sleep. We know this because her pulse continued to spike whilst knocked out. What we needed was an adrenalin blocker. So, we decided to try a tiny dose of the adrenalin-blocker propranolol. Dorothy started to improve. She found she could sit up for longer. After 20 years of speeding heart, especially in the morning, 10 mg meant she could get to 11 am and do all her jobs that needed her to be more upright. So, we tried a further hike and more improvements followed. From being bedbound for 20 years she managed a weekly excursion out without relapsing. She went on a cruise. She did some more research to read that adrenalin stimulated alpha receptors as well as beta receptors, and so we decided to add in an alpha-blocker, namely clonidine 25 mcg, building up to 200 mcg. Further improvement. Now, in the day, her maximum heart rate is 90 bpm and she is the best she has been in 25 years. The improved sleep achieved by the alpha- and beta-blockers was the mechanism by which Dorothy's 'wound' was able to heal, at long last.

A key point here is not to ignore your potential 'emotional hole'. It is all too easy to think that 'this doesn't affect me' without really considering it. Discovering and dealing with (as best as you can) whatever the issue is for you can release new energy for the good of your health and happiness.

> *But feelings can't be ignored, no matter how*
> *unjust or ungrateful they seem.*

The Diary of a Young Girl, Anne Frank, 1929 – 1945

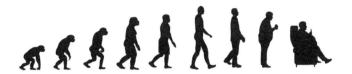

PART
4

GET YOUR ACT TOGETHER

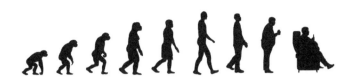

CHAPTER
15

GROUNDHOG DAYS

GETTING YOUR ACT TOGETHER:
A CHECK LIST

How well are you doing?

The starting point to prevent and treat all disease is exactly the same. Because I keep dragging my patients back to these basic subjects I call them Groundhog ABC (or rather, BAC – see below) interventions. This is remarkably difficult. People have come to expect that one symptom means one cause which means one drug to fix it. Big Pharma encourages this thinking because it makes for mindless medicine and big profits. Its propaganda has stuck in the Western psyche so that the perceived wisdom is that high-fat diets mean high cholesterol which means disease. *None* of these steps is correct. We now know that a high-fat PK diet extends quality and quantity of life. High fat is essential for optimum cholesterol since this is an essential raw material for healing and repair, the immune system and the brain.

- Groundhog Basic is the starting point for us all – see Appendix 2.

- Groundhog Acute is what we should all be doing in the event of acute infection – see Appendix 3.

- Groundhog Chronic is what we should do with any pathology and with increasing age – see Appendix 4.

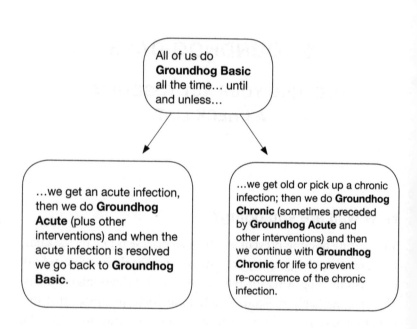

All of us do **Groundhog Basic** all the time… until and unless…

…we get an acute infection, then we do **Groundhog Acute** (plus other interventions) and when the acute infection is resolved we go back to **Groundhog Basic**.

…we get old or pick up a chronic infection; then we do **Groundhog Chronic** (sometimes preceded by **Groundhog Acute** and other interventions) and then we continue with **Groundhog Chronic** for life to prevent re-occurrence of the chronic infection.

Table 15.1 provides a reminder of the important interventions and what they achieve – the more you can do the healthier you will be and the longer you will live.

Ernest Hemingway (1899 – 1961) said this about love in *For Whom the Bell Tolls*: '*And another thing. Don't ever kid yourself about loving someone.*' As it is with love, so it is with (good) health – don't kid yourself.

How do we know we have done the Groundhogs sufficiently well for optimal health?

We so easily fool ourselves and think we have done a good job when in fact we have not. Addiction is the greatest blinding factor and tests often help us to see that which we do not wish to see.

However, while tests are useful, do not rely on standard reference ranges because these are established by looking at the blood tests of modern Westerners - who are not healthy! In Table 15.2 I list the ranges that I consider to be healthy. These are different from lab ranges which reflect the levels of 90% of the population. This is not an optimum health range since so many people no longer enjoy optimum health.

So, there you have it – two checklists, one to check that you have put in place the right interventions, and one to check that your test results indicate good health.

The modern checklist was born following the crash in 1935 of the prototype Boeing B-17 at Wright Field in Dayton, Ohio, where both pilots were killed. The concept of a pre-flight checklist was then introduced by Boeing. The investigation team had found that the pilots had forgotten to disengage the crucial gust locks (devices which stop control surfaces moving in the wind while parked) prior to take-off. Since then pre-flight checklists have grown in length and complexity – partly as a result of increasing technology and partly as a result of learning from crashes or errors. The statistics are impressive: '*By 2019, fatal accidents per million flights decreased 12 fold since 1970, from 6.35 to 0.51, and fatalities per trillion revenue passenger kilometre (RPK) decreased 81 fold from 3,218 to 40.*'[1] The above checklists are also in the name of reducing fatalities – yours!

This book is all about improving both the quantity and quality of your life. Its principles have been tried and tested on my willing and

Table 15.1: The benefits of the key interventions for good health

Intervention	Mitochondria	Thyroid Adrenals	Fermenting gut	Liver and kidney detox Antioxidants	Healing and repair	Emotional hole	Immuno-logical hole
The PK diet: go ketogenic (high fat and fibre; low carb and no sugar)	Fat, short-chain fatty acids (SCFAs) and ketones are the preferred fuel		Fibre gives us free energy. Fat requires minimal processing. (Sugar and starch risk fermentation)	Natural antioxidants in vegetables, berries and nuts	Essential raw materials	The adrenalin associated with metabolic syndrome makes us anxious (Carbs are addictive)	Essential raw materials (Sugar feeds infection)
The PK diet: go Paleo (no dairy or gluten grains)			(Milk and sugar can be fermented)		(Dairy increases the risk of osteoporosis)	(Dairy and wheat are addictive for some)	(Dairy and gluten are high risk for allergy and auto-immunity)
Sleep: time for healing and repair	Essential	Essential		Essential	Essential	Essential	Essential
Exercise	Increases numbers of mitochondria			Mobilises toxins	Builds muscle and bone		

	Warms and gives us free energy	Determines our circadian rhythm		Mobilises toxins from fat	Accelerates healing and repair	Makes us happy with free energy	Kills all infections
Sunshine	Warms and gives us free energy	Determines our circadian rhythm		Mobilises toxins from fat	Accelerates healing and repair	Makes us happy with free energy	Kills all infections
Basic package (see page 147)	Magnesium and other essentials	Essential raw materials		Multivitamins Minerals	Essential raw materials	Essential raw materials	Essential raw materials
Vitamin D					Prevents osteoporosis		Anti-inflammatory
Extra supplements	Co Q10 Vitamin B3 Acetyl-L-carnitine D ribose	Iodine Zinc Selenium Iron (Fe) Glandulars		Glutathione	Bone broth Silica Boron		
Vitamin C to bowel tolerance	Mops up free radicals from burning fuel	Vitamin C for steroid hormone synthesis	Kills upper gut fermenters	The master antioxidant	Raw material for connective tissue		Vitamin C kills all microbes (as does iodine)
Heating regimes: – FIR sauna – exercise + shower – hot bath with Epsom salts	Give us free energy			Mobilise toxins from fat	Improve circulation Reduce friction	The cooling down after encourages sleep	Kill all infections

ever-forgiving guinea-pig patients over that last 35+ years. Sometimes, I have stumbled around, but without my wonderful patients, I would not have been able to put together this roadmap to good health. My thanks go to them and my best wishes go to you, dear Reader.

Table 15.2: Healthy reference ranges for tests

Test	My healthy range	What it means	Action
Full blood count	Haemoglobin 130-145 g/l women 145-160 g/l men	Low means: anaemia; this will be either because you are losing blood OR you are not making it fast enough because you are deficient in a raw material or lacking the energy for manufacture	See a doctor for a faecal occult blood test to check for gut losses... And for faecal calprotectin both of which may indicate pathology Heavy periods? Test ferritin levels to check for iron deficiency
		High: Smoker? Polycythaemia rubra vera? Carbon monoxide poisoning?	Measure vitamin B12 Stop smoking and re-check Check appliances and install a carbon monoxide monitor See a doctor
	MCV (mean corpuscular volume) more than 95 fl	Either you are hypothyroid	You need to do thyroid function tests
		OR a poor methylator	Measure homocysteine. It is possible your GP can do this test. High homocysteine is a risk factor for fatigue but also arterial disease, cancer and dementia SO, this is an important test not least of all because if positive then we must screen all first-degree relative as high homocysteine runs in families

		Postal delay between blood taking and blood testing may cause a false macrocytosis (enlargement of red blood cells)	Check time between sample taking and testing
	MCV below 85 fl	Iron deficient? Thalassaemia?	Check ferritin
	WCC (white cell count) 4-6 x 10^{-3} ul	The normal range is positively skewed	Wait and repeat; if constantly high, look for a cause of inflammation
	WCC below 4 x 10^{-3} ul	White cells are being used up fast to fight infection AND/OR Lack of raw materials AND/OR Lack of energy to make white cells	Improve energy delivery mechanisms Improve nutritional status Identify the infection (see *The Infection Game*) – the commonest offenders in CFS are Epstein Barr virus ('mono'), Lyme and mycoplasma
	Neutrophils <3.2 x 10^9/l	High associated with bacterial infection	
	Lymphocytes <2 x 10^9/l	High associated with viral infection	
Neutrophil to lymphocyte ratio	>2.5	This points to inflammation...	...but this result does not tell us why. Inflammation is a major risk factor for cardiovascular disease
Platelet to lymphocyte ratio	>140	Ditto – inflammation	...but we know not why
ESR (eryth- rocyte sed- imentation rate)	below 5 mm/hour	Often the 'normal' lab range is up to 20! Again this means inflammation...	...but we know not why. Ditto above. Work out the why and re-check

Table 15.2: Healthy reference ranges for tests (cont.)

Test	My healthy range	What it means	Action
C reactive protein (CRP)	Less than 1 nm/l	Often the 'normal' lab range is said to be <5, but this is too high This is another inflammatory marker	If you are consuming carbs then you will be in a state of mild to moderate inflammation so adopt the PK diet
Total cholesterol	4.5-7.0 mmol/l for men 5.0-8.0 for women	Cholesterol is an essential raw material for all membranes, the brain and immune system. 'Desirable' ranges are set far too low to encourage doctors to prescribes statins. Too high a total cholesterol is a symptom of vitamin D deficiency and/or hypothyroidism	Address vitamin D deficiency: we should all be taking at least 5000 and up to 10,000 iu daily Test for thyroid hormone levels
		Too low is a major risk factor for psychiatric disease including depression – cholesterol is essential for the brain; high cholesterol protects against dementia; too low suggests over-dosing with statins or similar	Eat a PK high-fat diet
– Low density lipo-proteins (LDL)	3.0-4.5 mmol/l	LDL is an essential carrier to deliver cholesterol, phospholipids and triglycerides from the liver to cells for healing and repair; it is not a 'bad' fat. High LDL is inversely associated with mortality in most people over 60 years	Eat a PK high-fat diet

– Tri-glycerides	Less than 1 mmol/l (this must be a fasting sample)	Insulin brings down blood sugar by shunting it into storage as triglycerides; high triglycerides occur with high-carb diets	Eat a PK high-fat diet
HDL as a %age of total cholesterol (high-density lipoprotein, calculated by dividing HDL cholesterol by total	>40% of total cholesterol	If the percentage of the friendly HDL is low, this means HDL is being used up in the business of healing and repairing arteries – i.e. they are being damaged by something; this may be metabolic syndrome and/or high homocysteine and/or chronic inflammation	Put in place interventions then repeat test to check progress. The higher this result, the better – on a good PK diet I expect this to be 40%. A poor HDL %age is a symptom of arterial disease, not a cause
Electrolytes:			
– Sodium	139-142 mmol/l	If low this suggests lack of salt in the diet or losing salt due to diuretics or kidney failure	Adopt a PK diet – on a PK diet the need for salt increases – aim for 5 grams daily of Sunshine salt (page 150)
– Potassium	4.0-4.4 mmol/l	If very high this may be due to a delay in transport	Check time between sample taking and testing
	Below 4.0	Too little in diet	The body cannot store potassium – you have to eat it daily; there is plenty in a PK diet and Sunshine salt
– Serum mag-nesium	At least 0.8 mmol/l	Rarely done. Not a reliable test of body stores. Most doctors do not understand the difference between a serum magnesium and a red cell magnesium. Serum levels must be kept within a tight range, or the heart stops. Therefore, serum levels are maintained at the expense of red cell levels	If below 0.6 then you are in serious trouble and need urgent medical attention To correct take magnesium 300 mg daily and vitamin D 10,000 iu daily Improve energy delivery mechanisms

Table 15.2: Healthy reference ranges for tests (cont.)

Test	My healthy range	What it means	Action
– Creatinine	Below 115 umol/l	High protein diet and/ or high muscle mass Poor kidney function	Reduce protein intake and re-check Look for causes of kidney damage – glyphosate is one such
	Above 65 umol/l	Low protein diet and/ or low muscle mass Many CFS/ME patients have low creatinine as they have low muscle mass and cannot exercise	If there is no good reason for low muscle mass, then increase the protein intake
– Urea	4-7 mmol/l	High means dehydration May accompany high creatinine	You need water AND fat AND salt to be properly hydrated
– Uric acid	Below 320 umol/l (men) and 260 (women)	Uric acid is also a mycotoxin	If high, look for a fungal issue, possibly fermenting gut. Many anti-gout drugs work because they are antifungal
12-hour fasting glucose	Below 5.0 mmol/l	If higher you are starting to lose control of your blood sugar and are on the way to diabetes	Adopt a PK diet
Glyco-sylated haemo-globin	Less than 5.5% Less than 34 mmol/mol (Ranges have changed recently because nearly all Westerners eat too much carb and are on the way to diabetes)	A very useful test of average blood sugar over the previous three months. This is a great test of how well you are doing a PK diet	Adopt a PK diet and stick to it

		How does the NHS deal with this? By moving the goal posts. It is now considered acceptable to have a fasting glucose up to 7 mmol/l and a glycosylated Hb of 48	
Liver function tests:			
- GGT - AST - ALT	Below 20 U/l Below 20 U/l Below 20 U/l	If high then this is enzyme induction to deal with toxins, not liver damage	Look out for the source of the toxins: – from alcohol or other such drugs? – from toxins from the outside world? – from products of the upper fermenting gut?
– Alkaline phos-phatase	Below 80 U/l	If high suggests tissue damage, typically liver, gallbladder or bones	Find the cause
– LDH	Below 175	Ditto above. May also indicate muscle or heart damage I suspect where there are poor energy delivery mechanisms with early switch into anaerobic metabolism, this enzyme is induced	Find the cause Improve energy delivery mechanisms
– Bilirubin	Below 10 umol/l	Higher suggests poor detoxification via the glucuronide pathway so you will be more susceptible to toxic stress. When it is above 19 this is called Gilbert's syndrome	Identify the cause of the toxic stress and mitigate – see Chapter 13. Take glutathione 250 mg for life to improve liver detox. Since we live in a toxic world, I think we should all be taking this

Table 15.2: Healthy reference ranges for tests (cont.)

Test	My healthy range	What it means	Action
Bone: – Corrected calcium	2.35-2.45 mmol/l	Any lower suggests vitamin D deficiency. This is very common; we all need to take 5-10,000 iu daily	Sunshine salt has 5000 iu of vitamin D per 5 gram daily dose. Do not take calcium supplements – there is plenty in food - you just need to be able to absorb it with vitamin D. Too much calcium blocks magnesium absorption
		Normal 'bone markers' do not exclude osteoporosis	The best test for osteoporosis is a heel bone density scan which is accurate and involves no dangerous X-rays
Ferritin	100-250 pmol/l (for women) 150-350 pmol/l (for men and post-menopausal women) (Menstruating women run a lower ferritin level. Many doctors consider that a ferritin as low as 12 pmol/l is acceptable)	You are losing blood OR lacking iron (possibly due to lack of iron in the diet (meat) or malabsorption – you need an acid stomach to absorb iron. One cause of this is upper fermenting gut due to too much carb in the diet)	Adopt a PK diet Vitamin C to bowel tolerance
PSA (prostate specific antigen)	Age 40-49: up to 2.5 ng/ml Age 50-60: up to 3.5 ng/ml Age 60-70: up to 4.5 ng/ml ('ng/ml' and 'µg/l' are the same)	The PSA reflects the amount of prostate tissue; it is the rate of change that suggests malignancy	Do the PK diet – the growth promoters are carbs and dairy. Re-check at one-month intervals to see the rate of change

Vitamin B12	I like to see this above 1000 pg/ml ('Normal' ranges simply reflect the level which prevents pernicious anaemia)	You need more for optimum biochemistry	Sunshine salt has 5000 mcg per daily dose (the risible RDA for B12 is set at 1-3 mcg)
Homo-cysteine	I like to see this below 10 μmol/l (many lab reference ranges are less than 15)	High homocysteine means poor methylation. This is an essential biochemical tool to allow one to 'read' DNA, detoxify, synthesise enzymes and proteins and do much more Being a poor methylator is a MAJOR risk factor for arterial disease, dementia, cancer and degenerative disease	To normalise you need methylated B vitamins – that is to say, methyl B6 (pyridoxal 5 phosphate), methyl folate (methyl tetrahydrofolate) and methyl B12
Thyroid hormones:			
– TSH	I like to see this below 1.5 mU\l (The 'normal' range is negatively skewed. In the UK treatment is not given until the TSH is above 10)	A TSH tells us little but it is relied upon too heavily by many doctors to determine the dose of thyroid hormone.	See Chapter 8 plus our book *Ecological Medicine* for much more detail
– Free T4	I like to see this above 16 pmol/l		See Chapter 8 plus our book *Ecological Medicine* for much more detail

Table 15.2: Healthy reference ranges for tests (cont.)

Test	My healthy range	What it means	Action
	(My lab range is 12-22; some NHS ranges are 7-14. But some people do not feel well until running at 30 pmol/l)		
– Free T3	I like to see this above 4.0 pmol/l	Where there is thyroid hormone receptor resistance blood tests are misleading	See Chapter 8 See *Ecological Medicine* for much more detail
		If T3 is low compared with T4, this suggests poor conversion of inactive T4 to the active T3 – that is, T3 hypothyroidism	See Chapter 8 See *Ecological Medicine* for much more detail
– Reverse T3	10-24 ng/dl	A high level relative to the free T3 points to thyroid hormone receptor resistance – in this event the blood tests are not helpful	You must rely on the clinical picture to determine the dose of thyroid hormone. See *Ecological Medicine* for much more detail
– All		If TSH is high despite good levels of T4 and T3 then this points to thyroid hormone receptor resistance	See Chapter 8 See *Ecological Medicine* for much more detail

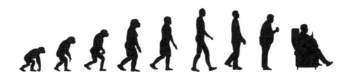

APPENDICES

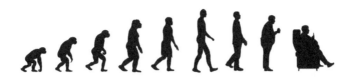

APPENDIX

1

THE PALEO-KETOGENIC (PK) DIET AND ESSENTIAL MICRONUTRIENTS

– MULTIVITAMINS, MINERALS, ESSENTIAL FATTY ACIDS

– WHAT TO EAT, WHICH SUPPLEMENTS TO TAKE

The Cure is in the Kitchen
Dr Sherry Rogers, environmental physician

The PK diet is non-negotiable. I spend more time talking about diet and cooking than all other subjects put together. Changing one's diet is the most difficult but the most important thing one needs to do for good health. There is much more detail of the WHY and the HOW in our books *Prevent and Cure Diabetes – delicious diets not dangerous drugs* and *The PK Cookbook – go paleo-ketogenic and get the best of both worlds*. Please do use them – they are born out of bitter experience.

Remember, outside of autumn/fall, primitive man ate a paleo-ketogenic diet and this would be largely comprised of raw meat and/

or raw fish and shellfish depending on where he lived. That was it. You may think this a boring diet, but boredom is secondary to survival. For some of the sickest patients, we have to return to this very primitive diet to allow them to recover. Natasha Campbell McBride describes this diet in her book *The GAPS Diet*.[1] An essential part of this diet is to access bone marrow. Perhaps this is what drove primitive man to using tools to smash open this treasure chest of fat and micronutrients and so the clever ones survived? Neanderthal man had a larger brain than modern man. As my patients often hear in the consulting room: 'My job is to get you well not to entertain you' (Yours Truly in *The PK Cookbook*. Some say that quoting oneself lacks humility. It is a good job then that Craig wrote the above paragraph!)

Guess what? I am not going to live my life eating raw meat and raw fish just so that I can live to a great age. We all have to work out a compromise diet that gets the best of both worlds. And that is going to be different for everyone and will change with age. For me, greed gets in the way – I love good food. So, we all need a starting point which can then be relaxed or tightened up on depending on age and disease state. Younger, healthy, physically active people can take more liberties than old, sick ones. I find myself in the old, healthy category and so I am still no paragon of virtue.

What to eat

This is a reasonable starting point for most. You can eat as much as you like of the following:

- Fats – saturated fats for energy such as lard, butter and ideally ghee (so long as you are sure you are not allergic to dairy – I am …. damnit), goose fat, coconut oil, palm oil.

- Oils – unsaturated fats which are also fuels but contain essential

148

omega-3 and -6 and beneficial omega-9 fatty acids. Hemp oil is ideal, containing the perfect proportion of omega 6 to omega 3 – that is, 4:1. These must be cold-pressed and not used for cooking or you risk 'flipping' them into toxic trans fats. Only cook with biochemically stable, saturated fats. (See our books *Prevent and Cure Diabetes – delicious diets not dangerous drugs* and T*he PK Cookbook – go paleo-ketogenic and get the best of both worlds* for more on good and bad fats.)

- Fibre (this is often included in the carb count of foods on packaging and leads to some confusion).

Also, foods that contain less than 5% carb, of which the most important are:

- Linseed – our *PK Cookbook* has a great recipe for linseed bread which looks and behaves like a small Hovis; linseed also makes a great base for muesli and porridge.

- Coconut cream – the Grace coconut milk is head and shoulders above all others with a 2% carb content. It is a great alternative to dairy.

- Brazil and pecan nuts are less than 5% carb.

- Salad – lettuce, cucumber, tomatos, peppers etc; avocado pear and olives (phew! I love them both).

- green leafy vegetables.

- mushrooms and fungi – a difficulty with this diet is eating enough fat; these foods are great for frying as they mop up delicious saturated fats.

- fermented foods (sauerkraut, kefir) – the carb content has been fermented out by microbes.

Care is needed with the following:

- meat, fish, shellfish and eggs – don't eat too much as excessive amounts can be converted back to carbohydrate. (See *The PK Cookbook* for details).

- Salt – 1 teaspoonful (5 grams) daily. Ideally use Sunshine salt, as below.

- Coffee and tea in moderation.

Take care with foods that are 5-10% carb (much more detail in T*he PK Cookbook*)

- Berries.

- Some nuts: almonds.

- Herbs and spices – these do have a carb content but in the small amounts normally used these are not going to spike blood sugar levels.

Avoid foods containing more than 10% carb as they switch on addictive eating. I know – I too am an addict.

- All grains, pulses, fruits (apart from berries and rhubarb) and their juices.

- Many nuts and seeds.

- Junk food, which is characterised by its high-carb content and addictive potential, including crisps (sorry, Craig).

- All dairy products except ghee.

- All sweeteners, natural or artificial, which simply switch on physical and psychological craving.

Supplements

Take micronutrient supplements for life to compensate for the deficiencies resulting from modern food production:

- A good multivitamin and multimineral. We need these simply because with Western agriculture there is a one-way movement of minerals from the soil, to plants, to animals and then to us humans. We throw them away. This lack of recycling means we are all deficient in such. (Once again, we discuss this in much more detail in *The PK Cookbook*, with referenced studies showing the result of this 'one-way' traffic.)

- I have got to the stage of my medical practice where I know exactly what must be done so I am now trying to make this as easy and inexpensive as possible. Consequently, I have put together 'Sunshine salt', which contains all essential minerals from sodium and selenium to magnesium and manganese, together with vitamins D 5000 iu and B12 5 mg in a 5-g/1 teaspoon dose. This does make life much easier. It tastes like a slightly piquant sea salt, can be used in cooking and means the rest of the family get a dose without realising it, especially all those men who believe they are immortal – aside from Craig that is, who was born a man and has had honorary womanhood bestowed upon him!

- Vitamin C – 5-15 g (yes, I mean 5000 to 15,000 mg, and, no, that is not a big dose) daily. (See Appendix 5 and our book *The Infection Game – life is an arms race* for the why.)

It is a shame that 'ichor' (the 'blood' of the Greek Gods which was said to retain the qualities of ambrosia, the food or drink of the gods, which gave them immortality, but which was deadly to mortals) does not seem to exist. And so, until ichor is found, or formulated, and made non-toxic to mortals, I shall 'eat PK', take my supplements and openly sprinkle Sunshine salt over my food.

Timing

Primitive man did not eat three regular meals a day, neither did he snack. Consultant neurologist Dale Bredesen reverses dementia with a PK diet but insists all daily food is consumed within a 10-hour window of time.[2] Once keto-adapted, you may feel a bit peckish and deserving of a snack, but the good news is that you will not get the associated 'energy dive' experienced by the carb addict who must eat according to the clock. Carb addicts feel a sudden loss of energy and HAVE to feed their addiction to get rid of this awful feeling. The keto-adapted do not experience this. A weekly 24-hour fast is also good for the metabolism. It may be counterintuitive, but the fact is that this enhances mental and physical performance.

If you have decided to go ahead with this diet, then believe me it is a bumpy ride. There is a whole new language to be learned. You will have to identify the glycogen sponge, anticipate the metabolic hinterland, get keto-adapted and prepare for detox and Herx reactions (see our books *Prevent and cure Diabetes – delicious diets not dangerous drugs* and *The PK Cookbook*. I simply cannot write all the nitty gritty detail here … at least get the *The PK Cookbook* which holds your intellectual hand through this difficult transition. Or just do it.)

Once established on the PK diet

The word 'doctor' comes from the Latin 'to teach'. I can show you the path, but you have to walk it. You have to become your own doctor. All diagnosis starts with hypothesis. We know the PK diet is the starting point to treat every disease and that is non-negotiable. Stick with this diet for life and it may be that this is all you have to do. Once PK is established you have to ask if you are functioning to your full physical and mental potential. Only you can know this.

If you are functioning to your full potential, then you can take the occasional liberty with your diet. Primitive man surely did. He did so in the autumn, although not with the high-carb foods that we can now access. Alcohol is a peculiar problem – it is addictive, high-carb and stimulates insulin directly. But I love alcohol – the jokes are so much funnier with a glass of cider on board and so I enjoy this occasional liberty at this stage in my life. I have to because Craig keeps sending me bottles of the most delicious cider… and I do not have the will power to tell him to stop. (Craig: 'Then I shall carry on. Luckily in return, I get delicious joints of pork and bacon.')

If you are *not* functioning to your full potential, then you must stick with the PK diet and re-read the rest of this book. Even if you do not experience immediate benefits, you will greatly increase your chance of a long and healthy life. It is a great consolation for me to be able to tell my CFS and ME patients that their best years are ahead of them.

The Chinese do not draw any distinction between food and medicine.

Lin Yutang (1895 – 1976) Chinese writer.
The Importance of Living
chapter 9, section 7.

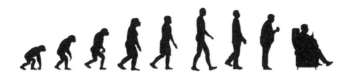

APPENDIX
2

GROUNDHOG BASIC

WHAT WE SHOULD ALL BE DOING
ALL THE TIME, ESPECIALLY KIDS

Because I constantly refer back to this basic approach, which is fundamental to the treatment of all infections, and by inference to the avoidance of the major killers (cancer, heart disease, dementia…) which are all driven by chronic infection, from here on I will call this 'Groundhog'. In the film *Groundhog Day*, this refers to a time loop as the same day repeats for the main protagonist, over and over. With the Groundhog approach to infection we have another sort of loop that bears constant repetition. The point here is that Groundhog done well will do much to prevent acute illness developing and chronic disease getting a foothold.

It is also the case that Groundhog will change through life as we are exposed to new infections and as our defences decline with age.

- All should do the Groundhog Basic all (well most) of the time

- All should be prepared to upgrade to Groundhog Acute to deal with unexpected and sudden infectious challenges. (Get your Groundhog Acute First Aid box stocked up now – see Appendix 3)

- All will need to move to Groundhog Chronic as we age and acquire an infectious load

It is so important to have all the above in place and then at the first sign of any infection take vitamin C to bowel tolerance (see Appendix 5) and use iodine for local infections, because:

- You will feel much better very quickly.

- Your immune system will not be so activated that it cannot turn off subsequently. So many patients I see with ME started their illness with an acute infection from which they never recovered – their immune system stayed switched on.

- The shorter and less severe the acute infection, the smaller the chance of switching on an inappropriate immune reaction, such as autoimmunity. Many viruses are associated with one type or another of arthritis – for example, 'palindromic rheumatism'.[†] I think of this as viral allergy.

- The shorter and less severe the acute infection, the smaller the chance the microbe concerned has of making itself a permanent home in your body. Many diseases, from Crohn's and cancer to polymyalgia and Parkinson's, have an infectious driver (see our book *The Infection Game*.

The supplements noted in Table A2.1 are what we have called the 'basic package' of supplements elsewhere in the book.

Table A2.1: Groundhog Basic

What to do	Notes
The Paleo-ketogenic diet – high fat, high fibre, very low carb – probiotic foods like kefir and sauerkraut – no dairy or grains – two meals a day with no snacking	See our books *Prevent and Cure Diabetes – delicious diets not dangerous drugs* for the WHY and *The PK Cookbook – go paleo-ketogenic and get the best of both worlds* for the HOW
A basic package of nutritional supplements – multi-vitamins, multi-minerals and vitamin D	A good multi-vitamin and Sunshine salt 1 tspn daily with food. 1 dsp hemp oil
Vitamin C	Dissolve 5 g vitamin C (ascorbic acid) in 500 ml mineral water and sip throughout the day; vitamin C has a short half life
Sleep 8-9 hours between 10:00 pm and 7:00 am	More in winter, less in summer
Exercise at least once a week when you push yourself to your limit	It is anaerobic exercise that produces lactic acid and stimulates the development of new muscle fibres and new mitochondria
Herbs, spices and fungi in cooking	Use your favourite herbs, spices and fungi in cooking and food, and lots of them – Yum yum!
If fatigue is an issue – address energy delivery mechanisms as best as you can	See our book *Diagnosing and Treating Chronic Fatigue Syndrome and Myalgic Encephalitis: it's mitochondria not hypochondria*
Heat and light	Keep warm; sunbathe at every opportunity
Use your brain	Foresight: Avoid risky actions like kissing,* unprotected sex Caution: Avoid vaccinations; travel with care Circumspection: Do not suppress symptoms with drugs; treat breaches of the skin seriously.

*Oscar Wilde (16 October 1854 – 30 November 1900) knew this, perhaps for different reasons than the risk of infection, when he wrote that: '*A kiss may ruin a human life.*'

(From *A Woman of No Importance* (is there ever such a thing? asks Craig))

†**Note**: Palindromic rheumatism is rheumatism that comes and goes. The word 'palindrome' was coined by English playwright Ben Johnson in the 17th Century from the Greek roots *palin* (πάλιν: 'again') and *dromos* (δρόμος; 'way, direction'). The first known palindrome, written as a graffito, and etched into the walls of a house in Herculaneum, reads thus: *sator arepo tenet opera rotas* – 'The sower Arepo leads with his hand the plough'. (idiomatic translation). Much of the graffiti (graffito is the singular of graffiti) found in Pompeii and Herculaneum are somewhat bawdy, some focusing on what the local ladies of the fine houses would like to do with certain named gladiators or, indeed, vice-versa… The authors leave it to the readers to do their own research.

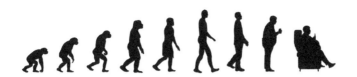

APPENDIX
3

GROUNDHOG ACUTE

WHAT WE SHOULD ALL DO AT THE FIRST SIGN OF ANY INFECTION, NO MATTER WHAT OR WHERE

At the first sign of any infection, you must immediately put in place Groundhog Acute. Do not forget the wise advice of Dr Fred Klenner (BS, MS, MD, FCCP, FAAFP, 1907 – 1984): *'The patient should get large doses of vitamin C in all pathological conditions while the physician ponders the diagnosis.'* Strike soon and strike hard because time is of the essence. I repeat myself here because it is so important:

- You will feel much better very quickly.

- Your immune system will not be so activated that it cannot turn off subsequently. So many patients I see with ME started their illness with an acute infection from which they never recovered – their immune system stayed switched on.

- The shorter and less severe the acute infection, the smaller the chance of switching on an inappropriate immune reaction, such as autoimmunity. Many viruses are associated with one type or another of arthritis – for example, 'palindromic rheumatism' (see page 158). I think of this as viral allergy.

- The shorter and less severe the acute infection, the smaller the chance the microbe concerned has of making itself a permanent home in your body. Many diseases, from Crohn's and cancer to polymyalgia and Parkinson's, have an infectious driver (see page 168 and our book *The Infection Game*).

At the first sign of the tingling, sore throat, runny nose, malaise, headache, cystitis, skin inflammation, insect bite, or whatever… Table A3.1 shows what you should do.

You may consider that doing all the above amounts to over-kill, but when that 'flu or coronavirus epidemic arrives,* as it surely will, you will be very happy to have been prepared and to have these weapons to hand so that you, your family, friends and neighbours will survive. Stock up your Groundhog Acute First Aid box now. As Lord Baden Powell wrote in *Scouting for Boys*, '*Be prepared*'; and heed the wisdom of Benjamin Franklin (17 January 1706 – 17 April 1790): '*By failing to prepare, you are preparing to fail.*'

The contents of the Groundhog Acute Battle First Aid box

John Churchill, 1st Duke of Blenheim (26 May 1650 – 16 June 1722), was a highly successful General, partly because he made sure his

*Footnote: Yes, this book was written before the arrival of Covid-19. Nostradamus, move over!

Table A3.1: Groundhog Acute

What to do	Why and How

The Paleo-ketogenic diet
– high fat, high fibre, very low carb
– probiotic foods like
  kefir and sauerkraut
– no dairy or grains
– two meals a day with
  no snacking
	See our books *Prevent and Cure Diabetes – delicious diets not dangerous drugs* for the WHY and *The PK Cookbook – go paleo-ketogenic and get the best of both worlds* for the HOW

You may consider a fast – this is essential for any acute gut infection. Drink rehydrating fluids – that is, Sunshine salt 5 g in 1 litre of water ad lib	*'Starve a cold; starve a fever'* (No, not a typo – starve any short-lived infection)
Vitamin C to bowel tolerance. The need for vitamin C increases hugely with any infection. Interestingly our bowel tolerance changes so one needs a much higher dose to get a loose bowel motion during an infection. If you do not have a very loose bowel motion within one hour of taking 10 g, take another 10 g. Keep repeating until you get diarrhoea. Most of us need 3-4 doses to abolish symptoms	Vitamin C greatly reduces any viral, or indeed any microbial, load in the gut (be aware that some of the infecting load of influenza virus will get stuck onto the sticky mucus which lines the lungs and is coughed up and swallowed). Vitamin C improves the acid bath of the stomach. Vitamin C protects us from the inevitable free-radical damage of an active immune system (see Appendix 5 for more detail.)
A good multi-vitamin Sunshine salt 1 tspn daily in water 1 dsp hemp oil	Sunshine salt in water because you should be fasting at a ratio of 5 g (1 tsp) in 1 l water to provide a 0.5% solution
Take Lugol's iodine 12%: 2 drops in a small glass of water every hour until symptoms resolve. Swill it round your mouth, gargle, sniff and inhale the vapour	It is well documented that 30 seconds of direct contact with iodine kills all microbes

Table A3.1: Groundhog Acute (cont.)

What to do	Why and How
With respiratory symptoms, put 4 drops of Lugol's iodine 12% into a salt pipe and inhale for 2 minutes; do this at least four times a day. Apply a smear of iodine ointment inside the nostrils	As above, 30 seconds of direct contact with iodine kills all microbes. This will contact-kill microbes on their way in or on their way out, rendering you less infectious to others
Apply iodine ointment 10% to any bite, skin break or swelling	Again, iodine contact-kills all microbes and is absorbed through the skin to kill invaders
Consume plenty of herbs, spices and fungi	If you are still struggling, then see *The Infection Game – life is an arms race* for effective herbal preparations and how to deal with complications of infection
Rest – listen to your symptoms and abide by them – sleep is even more important with illness	I see so many people who push on through acute illness and risk a slow resolution of their disease with all the complications that accompany such. The immune system needs the energy to fight! I find vitamin C to bowel tolerance combined with a good night's sleep has kept me cold free and flu free for 35 years
Heat – keep warm	Fevers kill all microbes. Some people benefit from sauna-ing. Do not exercise!
Light – sunshine is best	Sunbathe if possible
Use your brain – do not suppress symptoms with drugs	Symptoms of infection help the body fight infection. Anti-inflammatory drugs inhibit healing and repair – they allow the microbes to make themselves permanently at home in the body
If you develop other acute symptoms…	…see *The Infection Game – life is an arms race* But all treatments start with Groundhog Acute.

Table A3.2: What to keep in your **Battle First Aid box**

When	What
For acute infections	Vitamin C as ascorbic acid at least 500 g (it is its own preservative so lasts for years) Lugol's iodine 15% – at least 50 ml (it is its own preservative so lasts for years)
Conjunctivitis, indeed, any eye infection	Iodine eye drops e.g. Minims povidine iodine 5% OR 2 drops of Lugol's iodine 15% in 5 ml of water; this does not sting the eyes and is the best killer of all microbes in the eye
Upper airway infections	Lugol's iodine – to be used in steam inhalation, OR Salt pipe into which drizzle 4 drops of Lugol's iodine 15% per dose
Skin breaches	Salt – 2 tsp (10 g) in 500 ml water (approx 1 pint) plus 20 ml Lugol's iodine 15%. Use ad lib to wash the wound. Once clean, allow to dry and then smother with iodine oil (coconut oil 100 ml with 10 ml of Lugol's iodine 15% mixed in) . Plaster or micropore to protect
Fractures	If the skin is broken – as for Skin breaches above Immobilise If the limb is fractured, wrap in cotton wool to protect and bandage abundantly with vet wrap to splint it Next stop... casualty
Burns	As for skin breaches above If a large burn, then use cling film to protect once cleaned (put the iodine ointment on the cling film first, then apply to the burn) Protect as per fracture above. For a very large burn... next stop casualty
All injuries involving skin breaches	Sterile dressings: Melolin is a good all-rounder Large roll of cotton wool Crêpe bandages (various sizes) Micropore tape to protect any damaged area from further trauma Vet wrap bandage – this is wonderful stuff, especially if you are in the wilds, to hold it all together

Table A3.2: What to keep in your **Battle First Aid box (cont.)**

When	What
Gastroenteritis	Sunshine salt: To make up a perfect rehydration drink mix 5 g (1 tsp) in 1 litre of water to give a 0.5% solution
Urine infections	Multistix to test urine D-mannose: One typical product is Now Foods D-Mannose (available from iHerb), 500 mg, 120 veg capsules – take 3 x 500 mg capsules one to three times a day Potassium citrate: some example products with their respective doses are: • Effervescent tablets (brand Effercitrate) – take two tablets, up to three times a day, dissolved into a whole glassful of water. • Liquid medicine (brand Cymaclear) – take two x 5 ml spoonfuls, stirred into a whole glassful of water. You can take up to three doses a day. • Sachets (brand Cystopurin) – empty the contents of one sachet into a whole glassful of water. Stir it well before drinking. Take one sachet, three times daily
Bacterial infections	Consider acquiring antibiotics for intelligent use. These should not be necessary if you stick to Groundhog Basic and apply Groundhog Acute BUT I too live in the real world and am no paragon of virtue, so, if you slip off the band wagon:
– Dental	Amoxil 500 mg x 21 capsules
– ENT and respiratory	Cephalexin 500 mg three times daily
– Diverticulitis	Doxycycline 100 mg twice daily (DO NOT USE IN PREGNANCY OR FOR CHILDREN)
– Urinary	Trimethoprim 200 g twice daily
– Any	If you are susceptible to a particular infection, then make sure you always hold the relevant antibiotic; the sooner you treat, the less the damage, but always start with Groundhog Acute

armies were fully equipped for battle. The essence of success is to be prepared with the necessary to combat all assailants. As I have said, strike early and strike hard. Of John Churchill, Captain Robert Parker (who was at the Battle of Blenheim, 13 August 1704) wrote: '...*it cannot be said that he ever slipped an opportunity of fighting....*' We must be equally belligerent in our own individual battles. Part of this belligerence is preparedness, so keep the following in your own 'Battle First Aid Box' and use it at the first sign of attack.

Putting together such a Battle First Aid Box is as much an intellectual exercise as a practical one and this book, along with our books *The Infection Game – life is an arms race* and *Prevent and Cure Diabetes – delicious diets, not dangerous drugs* give such intellectual imperative. As Shakespeare writes in *Henry V*: '*All things are ready, if our mind be so.*'

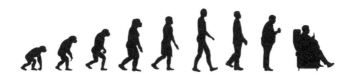

APPENDIX

4

GROUNDHOG CHRONIC

WHAT WE SHOULD ALL BE DOING INCREASINGLY AS WE AGE TO LIVE TO OUR FULL POTENTIAL

As we age, we acquire infections. My DNA is comprised 15% of retro virus. So is yours. I was inoculated with Salk polio vaccine between 1957 and 1966 so I will probably have simian virus 40, a known carcinogen. I am probably carrying the chickenpox, measles, mumps and rubella viruses because I suffered those as a child. I was also a bit spotty so proprionibacterium acnes may be a potential problem. At least 90% of us have been infected with Epstein Barr virus. I have been bitten by insects and ticks from all over the British Isles so I could also be carrying Lyme (borrelia), babesia and perhaps others. I have been a cat owner and could well test positive for bartonella. I have suffered several fractures which have healed but I know within that scar issue will be lurking some microbes – feed them some sugar and they will multiply and give me arthritis. I have had dental abscesses in the past and have one root filling which undoubtably will also harbour microbes. In the past, I have consumed a high carb diet which inevitably results in fermenting gut. On the good side, my puritanical upbringing means I have been free from STDs (thank you Mum!).

All these microbes have the potential to drive nasty diseases such as leukaemia, lymphoma, dementia, Parkinson's, heart disease, auto-immunity, cancer and so on. See '*The Infection Game – life is an arms race*' for more detail on this. I cannot eliminate them from my body, I have to live with them. I too am part of the Arms Race of the aforementioned book! Of course, this is a race I will (eventually) lose, but I will settle for losing it when I am 120. I am hoping that Groundhog Chronic will handicap my assailants and stack the odds in my favour.

So, as we age and/or we acquire stealth infections (see T*he Infection Game – life is an arms race*), we all need Groundhog Chronic. It is an extension of Groundhog Basic. Most will end up doing something between the two according to their health and history. But as you get older you have to work harder to stay well.

> "*Youth is wasted on the young*"
> Oscar Wilde (1854-1900)

If you are tiring from Groundhog, be inspired by these quotations:

> *We are what we repeatedly do. Excellence, then, is not an act, but a habit.*
> Idiomatic translation by Will Durrant in *The Story of Philosophy* of the Ancient Greek original:

> *Excellence is an art won by training and habituation…*
> Aristotle, 384 BC – 322 BC

> *repetitio est mater studiorum* – 'repetition is the mother of all learning'
> Old Latin Proverb

Table A4.1: Groundhog Chronic

What to do	Why	What I do
		My patients always ask me what I do. I am no paragon* of virtue, but I may have to become one eventually!
The Paleo-ketogenic (PK) diet – high fat, high fibre, very low carb. Probiotic foods like kefir and sauerkraut. No dairy or grains. Two meals a day and no snacking. Source the best quality foods you can find and afford – organic is a great start!	See our books *Prevent and Cure Diabetes – delicious diets not dangerous drugs* for the WHY and *The PK Cookbook – go paleo-ketogenic and get the best of both worlds* for the HOW	Yes. I do the PK diet 95% of the time. Glass of cider at weekends! Other liberties if eating out or socialising. But my friends are all becoming PK adapted too!
Eat daily food within a 10-hour window of time...	...so 14 hours a day when stomach is empty – this keeps the stomach acid and so decreases the chances of microbes invading. Maintains ketosis.	Nearly there... breakfast at 8:00 am, supper 6.30 pm
Consider episodic fasting one day a week	This gives the gut a lovely rest and a chance to heal and repair	I do this some weeks. The trouble is I am greedy and love food!
A basic package of nutritional supplements – multi-vitamins, multi-minerals and vitamin D		A good multi-vitamin and Sunshine salt 1 tspn daily with food 1 dsp hemp oil
Glutathione 250 mg daily Iodine 25 mg weekly	We live in such a toxic world we are inevitably exposed. Glutathione and iodine are helpful detox molecules (some people do not tolerate iodine in high doses)	Yes

Table A4.1: Groundhog Chronic (cont.)

What to do	How and Why	What I do
Vitamin C to 90% of bowel tolerance (BT); dissolve your bowel-tolerance amount in mineral water and sip throughout the day. Vitamin C has a short half life. Remember BT will change with age, diet and circumstance	With age, influenza becomes a major killer. With Groundhog you need never even get it!	I currently need 8 grams in 24 hours BUT I never get colds or influenza that last more than 24 hours
Lugol's iodine 15% 2 drops daily in water	Swill round the mouth and swallow last thing at night	Yes
Make sure your First Aid box is stocked	So, you have all your ammo to hand to hit new symptoms hard and fast	Yes – even when I go away, I take this – often to treat sickly others!
Sleep 8-9 hours between 10:00 pm and 7:00 am Regular power nap in the day	More in winter, less in summer Good sleep is as vital as good diet	Yes
Exercise within limits. By this I mean you should feel fully recovered next day. If well enough, once a week push those limits, so you get your pulse up to 120 beats per min and all your muscles ache. It is never too late to start!	No pain no gain. Muscle loss is part of ageing – exercise slows this right down Helps to physically dislodge microbes from their hiding places (I suspect massage works similarly)	Yes. Thankfully I am one of those who can and who enjoys exercise
Take supplements for the raw materials for connective tissue such as glucosamine. Bone broth is the best!	With age we become less good at healing and repair	Yes

Herbs, spices and fungi in cooking	Use your favourite herbs, spices and fungi in cooking and food, and lots of them!	Yes... Because I love food!
Consider herbs to improve the defences – see *The Infection Game: life is an arms race*	Astragalus, cordyceps and rhodiola	Sometimes when in stock and I remember
Address energy delivery mechanisms as below	See our book *Diagnosing and treating Chronic fatigue syndrome and myalgic encephalitis: it's mitochondria not hypochondria*	Yes Craig – I've got the book![†]
Take the mitochondrial package of supplements daily vis: CoQ10 100 g, niacinamide slow release 1500 mg, acetyl-L-carnitine 500 mg. D ribose 5-10 grams at night if you have really overdone things	With age fatigue becomes an increasing issue because our mitochondrial engines start to slow. The ageing process is determined by mitochondria. Look after them!	Yes with the exception of carnitine because I eat meat and my digestion is good
Mitochondria may be going slow because of toxins – consider tests of toxic load to see if you need to do any detox	A good all-rounder is Genova urine screen with DMSA 15 mg per kg of body weight. You can get this test through https://naturalhealthworldwide.com/	This is the only test I have ever done on myself! It showed background levels of toxic minerals
Check your living space for electromagnetic pollution	You can hire a detection meter from Healthy House www.healthy-house.co.uk/electro/meters-and-monitors	Yes. The cordless phone has gone! I never hold a mobile phone to my ear – I use the speaker Turn wifi off at night

Table A4.1: Groundhog Chronic (cont.)

What to do	How and Why	What I do
Review any prescription medication – they are all potential toxins The need for drugs is likely to be symptomatic of failure to apply Groundhog	Ask yourself why you are taking drugs? See our book *Ecological Medicine*. Once Groundhog is in place many drugs can be stopped. Taking prescription drugs is the fourth commonest cause of death in Westerners	I never take symptom-suppressing medication. This has allowed full and now pain-free recovery from three broken necks (horses again) and other fractures
Consider tests of adrenal and thyroid function since these glands fatigue with age and chronic infection	Thyroid bloods tests and adrenal saliva tests available through https://naturalhealthworldwide.com/ Core temperatures are help-ful for fine-tuning adrenal and thyroid function with glandulars. See Chapter 8	I find glandulars very helpful and currently take thyroid glandular 60 mg in the morning and 30 mg midday Adrenal glandular 500 mg once daily
Heat and light	Always keep warm. Sunbathe at every opportunity. Holidays in warm climates with sunbathing and swimming are excellent for killing infections and detoxing	I am a pyromaniac! My kitchen is lovely and warm with a wood-fired range. I work in my conservatory with natural light. I sunbathe as often as wet Wales permits. Do not forget hyperthermia and light as a good treatment for chronic infections – see Chapter 11
Use your brain	Foresight: Avoid risky actions like kissing, unprotected sex. Caution: Avoid vaccinations. Choose travel destinations with care. Circumspection: Do not symptom-suppress with drugs; treat breaches of the skin seriously.	I have to say that with age this is much less of an issue! No vaccinations. No foreign travel except to the Continent to see my daughter and to do lectures.

onsuetudinis magna vis est – the force of habit is great
Cicero, 106 BC – 43 BC

(Assassinated for his opposition to Mark Antony, Cicero's last words were purportedly, 'There is nothing proper about what you are doing, soldier, but do try to kill me properly.')

*The English noun 'paragon' (see page 169) comes from the Italian word *paragone*, which is a touchstone – a black stone that is used to tell the quality of gold.

Sarah has commented thus: 'Yes, Craig – I've got the book!' This is a reference to our consultations. Often Sarah is heard to say (in answer to my many questions): 'It's in that book, the one you wrote,' to which I answer: 'Yes, Sarah – I've got the book!'.

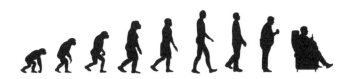

APPENDIX
5

VITAMIN C

LEARN TO USE THIS VITAL TOOL WELL:
THE KEY IS GETTING THE DOSE RIGHT

Vitamin C is a fantastically useful tool and in recent years has revolutionised my practice. It is the starting point to treat upper fermenting gut and all infections acute and chronic and therefore any condition involving inflammation. It multitasks to improve detoxing, is an essential antioxidant and is vital for healing and repair. It kills all microbes (bacteria, viruses and fungi) and is toxic to cancer cells. In healthy people, it slows the ageing process; in the acute and chronically sick, vitamin C to bowel tolerance is part of Groundhog Acute and Chronic described in this book. In achieving all this, vitamin C is completely non-toxic to human cells. There is much more detail in our book *The Infection Game – life is an arms race* but I will provide the basics here.

Vitamin C was the final tool that allowed me to tell my patients that vaccination was redundant since we had a far more effective, and far safer, tool in vitamin C. With vitamin C we get the best of both worlds: children can safely experience viral infections without risking complications of such, but receive the vital, live-virus immune programming needed to protect against disease later in life, particularly cancer.* The only vaccination I recommend is tetanus, but this should be postponed until the child is at risk of stabbing a muck-caked pitchfork through her foot.† And yes, I have done that too.

The key to vitamin C is the dose. We simply do not take enough of the stuff. The reason is to be found in Nature – all other animals (except guinea pigs and fruit bats and dry-nosed primates) can synthesise their own vitamin C. Furthermore, the amount generated is matched to requirements – vitamin C synthesis is hugely ramped up to deal with infection. Goats, for example, may generate 15 grams a day on demand. We humans have lost this essential biochemical function but instead we have our brains. So, use them! (For the genetics of vitamin C synthesis see Drouin et al, 2011[3])

*Footnote: Why does experiencing viral infections when a child protect against cancer in later life? We now know that getting an acute febrile (with a fever) illness as a child reduces overall cancer risk, and the more often this occurs, the better. At the very least children should get rubella and chickenpox (vaccination is no substitute), which are the most protective against cancer, but so too are infections with measles, mumps, pertussis (whooping cough) and scarlet fever.[1, 2] Researchers Hoption Cann et al conclude that: 'Infections may play a paradoxical role in cancer development with chronic infections often being tumorigenic and acute infections being antagonistic to cancer.'

†Note from Craig: My 'tetanus moment' was whilst climbing a tree at my Nan's. I was reaching to a bird's nest and fell. A strategically placed rusty nail (holding a swing) ripped down my chest from just under the neck to near the tummy button. If you look carefully, you can still see a scar. It is only the second time I ever saw my Nan cry. We went to the hospital for the vaccination. I was over the moon because I had a scar to show off to my school friends.

Thankfully we have a mechanism to determine the dose we require. This will need to be varied from day to day because the body absorbs what it needs and leaves the excess in the gut. This allows us to adjust the dose according to our guts. Turn this logic on its head – the dose required to achieve bowel tolerance is a reflection of our total infectious load, the extent to which we have a fermenting gut as well as our toxic load and possibly other issues. In other words, our bowel tolerance is a measure of our health – or lack of it.

Lower bowel tolerance => healthier
Higher bowel tolerance => unhealthier

How to take vitamin C to bowel tolerance

- Do the PK diet – vitamin C is much better absorbed in the absence of sugar and starch. There is no point killing microbes with vitamin C if you are feeding them at the same time.

- Take ascorbic acid at least twice daily (could be more often). It dissolves much better in warm water. Add fizzy water to produce a rather delicious drink. The ascorbic acid helps to sterilise the upper gut and prevents fermentation of food there. Any microbes inadvertently consumed with foods are killed. Acid further helps us digest proteins and also helps the absorption of essential minerals, such as iron and zinc

- Use ascorbic acid, which is the cheapest and most effective form of vitamin C. If this is not tolerated, then use a neutral preparation such as sodium or magnesium ascorbate. Once you are PK and vitamin C-adapted, you should tolerate ascorbic acid well. The cheapest form of ascorbic acid is fermented from corn but anyone with a corn allergy may not tolerate this at all. Failing that, one can (with some effort) get ascorbic acid from sago palm, tapioca or beet.

- Start with 2 grams twice daily and increase at the rate of 1 gram every day. You will start to get foul smelling wind. This occurs initially as microbes in the upper gut are killed, swept downstream and fermented by microbes in the lower gut. Later it occurs as you start to kill some of the friendlies in the lower gut. This is likely to need more than 10 grams of vitamin C per day. Keep increasing the dose until you get diarrhoea. Hold the dose at this level for 24 hours. At this point you should have a clean, digesting (non-fermenting) upper gut with low levels of microbes in the lower gut.

- Adjust the daily dose in the longer term. The idea is to find a dose of vitamin C that kills the grams of unfriendly microbes in the upper gut but does not kill the kilograms of friendly microbes in the lower gut. This will depend on several variables that you will have to work out for yourself vis, to find a dose that:

  - allows you to pass a normally formed daily turd

  - produces no smelly farting

  - stops you getting coughs, colds and flu when all around are succumbing

  - reduces, gets rid of or reverses any disease symptoms that you may be suffering from. These may be symptoms of upper fermenting gut or of chronic infection. As you can see from the Cathcart link below, you have to get to 90% of bowel tolerance to reverse the symptoms of any disease process.

At the first hint of any infection, such as a tickle in the throat, runny nose, sneeze, cough, feeling unwell, headache, cystitis... Well, you know what from bitter experience:

- Immediately take 10 grams of vitamin C. (half this dose for children, according to body weight). If this does not produce diarrhoea within one hour, then

- Take another 10 grams. If this does not produce diarrhoea within one hour, then

- Take another 10 grams... and so on. Some people need 200 g to get a result. Whilst this may seem like a huge dose, compare this with sugar – four bars of milk chocolate would provide a similar dose of sugar, and vitamin C is legions safer than sugar!

Some people are appalled at the idea of vitamin C causing diarrhoea, but I have to say I would rather have a jolly good bowel emptying crap than suffer the miserable symptoms of flu or a cold for the next two weeks. Indeed, I have not suffered such for 35 years thanks to vitamin C. My father used to say, 'You can't beat a good shit, shave and shampoo'.

Adjust the frequency and timing of subsequent doses to maintain wellness. Remember the dose is critical. You cannot over-dose; you can only under-dose. Just do it!

I am not alone in this advice, as is shown by the work of Robert Cathcart.

Dr Robert Cathcart

Dr Cathcart was a similar advocate of high-dose vitamin C. Some helpful clinical details can be seen at the website of the Vitamin C Foundation: http://vitamincfoundation.org/www.orthomed.com/titrate.htm[4]

Key points of the Vitamin C Foundation paper are:

- Everyone's bowel tolerance dose is unique to them. It will vary through time with age, diet and infectious load. You have to work it out for yourself and it will not remain constant.

- You must get to 80-90% of your bowel tolerance dose for vitamin C to relieve symptoms. This is another useful clinical tool as you can feel so much better so very quickly if you use vitamin C properly.

Cathcart details many diseases that are improved with vitamin C. Interestingly this includes many cases of arthritis. I suspect this illustrates one mechanism of arthritis, which is that it is often driven by allergy to gut microbes. Correct this by eliminating the upper-gut microbes and the arthritis goes. For example, we know ankylosing spondylitis is an inflammation driven by *Klebsiella* in the gut and rheumatoid arthritis is driven by *Proteus mirabilis*.

Dr Paul Marik

From the Eastern Virginia Medical School in Norfolk, Virginia, Marik added intravenous vitamin C to his normal antibiotic protocol for treating patients diagnosed with advanced sepsis and septic shock in his intensive care unit. Before using vitamin C, the mortality was 40%. Mortality is now less than 1%. Had this been a novel antibiotic it would have made headline news.

Dr Marik offered the following observations: 'In the doses used, vitamin C is absolutely safe. No complications, side effects or precautions. Patients with cancer have safely been given doses up to 150 grams - one hundred times the dose we give. In the patients with renal impairment we have measured the oxalate levels; these have all been in the safe range. Every single patient who received the protocol had an improvement in renal function.[5]

(Please note that anyone receiving intravenous vitamin C must be first checked for glucose-6-phosphate dehydrogenase deficiency. High-dose vitamin C in these people may cause a haemolytic anaemia. I can find no evidence of this being an issue for oral vitamin C.)

There is lots more good science and practical detail at *AscorbateWeb*.[6]

And if nothing else, please do remember that 'vitamin C' is Spanish for 'vitamin Yes'!

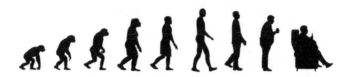

REFERENCES

Chapter 6: How the body generates energy for life

1. Inglis-Arkell E. 10 Scientists who experimented on themselves. *Gizmodo* 25 February 2011. (https://io9.gizmodo.com/10-scientists-who-experimented-on-themselves-5769654 - accessed 12 May 2020)

2. Bredesen DE, Amos EC, Ahdidan J. Reversal of cognitive decline in Alzheimer's disease. *Aging* 2016; 8(6): 1250-1258. www.ncbi.nlm.nih.gov/pmc/articles/PMC4931830/

3. Nishihara K. Disclosure of the major causes of mental illness – mitochondrial deterioration in the brain neurons via opportunistic infection. *Journal of Biological Physics and Chemistry* 2012; 12: 11-18.

Chapter 7: Energy delivery – the mitochondrial energy

1. Myhill S, Booth N, McLaren-Howard J. Chronic fatigue syndrome and mitochondrial dysfunction. *International Journal of Clinical and Experimental Medicine* 2009; 2: 1-16. (www.ijcem.com/files/IJCEM812001.pdf).

2. Booth N, Myhill S, McLaren-Howard J. Mitochondrial dysfunction and pathophysiology of myalgic encephalomyelitis/chronic fatigue syndrome (ME/CFS). *International Journal of Clinical and Experimental Medicine* 2012; 5(3): 208-220 (www.ijcem.com/files/IJCEM1204005.pdf).

3. Myhill S, Booth NE, McLaren-Howard J. Targeting mitochondrial

dysfunction in the treatment of myalgic encephalomyelitis/chronic fatigue syndrome (ME/CFS) – a clinical audit. *International Journal of Clinical and Experimental Medicine* 2013; 6(1): 1-15. (www.ijcem.com/files/IJCEM1207003.pdf).

Chapter 9: Sleep

1. Halberg F, Cornelissen G, Katinas G, Syutkina EV, et al. Transdisciplinary unifying implications of circadian findings in the 1950s. *Journal of Circadian Rhythms* 2003; 1: Article 2. http://doi.org/10.1186/1740-3391-1-2
2. *The Boke of Saint Albans* https://archive.org/stream/bokeofsaintalban00bern/bokeofsaintalban00bern_djvu.txt (accessed 5 July 2020)

Chapter 13: Energy expenditure – the immunological hole in the energy bucket

1. Kyle S. The science behind 'man flu' *Br Med J* 2017; 359: j5560. doi: https://doi.org/10.1136/bmj.j5560
2. Sedghy F, Varasteh A-R, Moghadam M. Interaction between air pollutants and pollen grains: The role on the rising trend in allergy. *Rep Biochem Mol Biol* 2018; 6(2): 219–224. www.ncbi.nlm.nih.gov/pmc/articles/PMC5941124/
3. Derry D. Iodine: the forgotten weapon against influenza viruses. *Thyroid Science* 2009; 4(9): R1-R5.
4. Brewer J, Thrasher JD, Hooper D. Chronic illness associated with mold and mycotoxins: is naso-sinus fungal biofilm the culprit? *Toxins* 2014; 6(1): 66-80. www.ncbi.nlm.nih.gov/pmc/articles/PMC3920250/
5. Tuuninen T, Rinne KS. Severe sequelae to mold-related illness as demonstrated in two Finnish cohorts. *Front Immunol* 2017. doi.org/10.3389/fimmu.2017.00382

Chapter 14: Energy expenditure – the emotional hole in the energy bucket

1. Raveraa S, Panfoli I, Calziaa D, Aluigi MG, Bianchini P, Diaspro A, Mancardi G, Morelli A. Evidence for aerobic ATP synthesis in isolated myelin vesicles. *International Journal of Biochemistry & Cell Biology* 2009; 41: 1581–1591. https://pubmed.ncbi.nlm.nih.gov/19401152/

2. Dunbar RIM, Sosis R. Optimising human community sizes *Evolution and Human Behavior* 2018; 39(1): 106-111. www.ncbi.nlm.nih.gov/pmc/articles/PMC5756541/

Chapter 15: Groundhog Days – getting your act together

1. Aviation safety. https://en.wikipedia.org/wiki/Aviation_safety

Appendix 1: The PK diet

1. Campbell-McBride N. *Gut and Psychology Syndrome*.2E. Medinform Publishing, 2018.

2. Bredesen DE. Reversal of cognitive decline: a novel therapeutic program. *Aging* 2014; 6(9): 707-717. (www.drmyhill.co.uk/drmyhill/images/0/07/Reversal-of-Cognitive-decline-Bredesen.pdf)

Appendix 5: Vitamin C

1. Zandvliet HA, Wel Evd. Science: Increase in cancer cases as a consequence of eliminating febrile infectious diseases. Nederlandse Vereniging Kritisch Prikken www.wanttoknow.info/health/cancer_link_vaccination_fever_research.pdf. (This includes reference 54 medical papers.)

2. Hoption Cann SA, Netten JPv, Netten Cv. Acute infections as a means of cancer prevention: opposing effects to chronic infections? *Cancer Detect Prev* 2006; 30(1): 83-93. www.ncbi.nlm.nih.gov/pubmed/16490323

3. Drouin G, Godin J-R, Page B. The genetics of vitamin C loss in vertebrates. *Current Genomics* 2011; 12(5): 371-378. www.ncbi.nlm. nih.gov/pmc/articles/PMC3145266/-

4. Cathcart RF. Vitamin C, titrating to bowel tolerance, anascorbemia, and acute induced scurvy. *Medical Hypotheses* 1981; 7: 1359-1376. http://vitamincfoundation.org/www.orthomed.com/titrate.htm

5. Levy TE. Vitamin C and sepsis – The genie is now out of the bottle. *Orthomolecular Medicine News Service* 24 May 2017. http://ortho-molecular.activehosted.com/index.php?action=social&chash=-44f683a84163b3523afe57c2e008bc8c.66

6. Reviews, Letters, Surveys, Editorials and Related Issues *Ascorbate Web* http://seanet.com/~alexs/ascorbate/index.htm#Rev-Ed (accessed 7 June 2020)

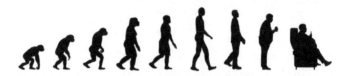

RESOURCES

Natural Health Worldwide
https://naturalhealthworldwide.com

Testing laboratories

No practitioner referral is needed for these:

> https://aonm.org
> https://medichecks.com
> www.mineralstate.com
> www.btsireland.com/joomla/
> https://smartnutrition.co.uk/health-tests/
> https://thriva.co

These laboratories require a practitioner referral:

> www.gdx.net/uk
> www.doctorsdata.com
> www.greatplainslaboratory.com
> www.biolab.co.uk

The Healthy House Ltd
www.healthy-house.co.uk
Tel: +44 (0)845 450 5950
Tel from a mobile: +44 (0)1453 752216

Supplement resources

D-mannose

One typical product is:
https://uk.iherb.com/pr/Now-Foods-DMannose-500-mg-120-Veggie-
    Caps/525
– take 3 x 500 mg capsules one to three times a day

Iodine

Lugol's iodine 12% can be obtained from
www.amazon.co.uk/Lugols-Iodine-12-Solution-30ml/dp/B00A25GCLO
and Lugol's iodine 15% can be obtained from
www.salesdrmyhill.co.uk/lugols-iodine-15-463.p.asp

Sunshine salt

One teaspoon (5 grams) contains all the minerals and vitamin D
needed for one day
www.salesatdrymyhill.co.uk/sunshine-salt-300-g-392-p.asp

Vitamins and non-herbal supplements

    UK   www.salesatdrmyhill.co.uk
    UK   www.biocare.co.uk
    UK   www.naturesbest.co.uk
    USA   www.swansonvitamins.com
    USA   www.purtan.com

Herbs

    UK   www.indigo-herbs.co.uk
    UK   ww.hydridherbs.co.uk
    USA   www.mountainroseherbs.com

INDEX

Note *fn* signifies 'footnote'.

Note *fn* signifies 'footnote'.

Note *fn* signifies 'footnote'.

Note *fn* signifies 'footnote'.